# SAVVY EATING
## FOR THE
# WHOLE FAMILY

# DISCLAIMER

The information contained in this book is intended as a guideline and inspiration for families who want to enjoy eating well. It is not a substitute for your own doctor's advice. In particular, the specific dietary needs of infants and individuals with various medical conditions are topics too specific for a book of this nature.

While every effort has been made to clearly and accurately present the most current knowledge on nutrition, interpretation, and application of Savvy Eating guidelines varies from person to person. As the reader, it is your responsibility to consult with your doctor and the doctors who care for your family before making any major changes in your family's diet.

# SAVVY EATING
## FOR THE
# WHOLE FAMILY

*Whole Foods, Whole Family, Whole Life*

## Margaret McCullers Kocsis, M.D.

CAPITAL SAVVY SERIES

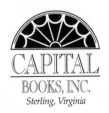

CAPITAL
BOOKS, INC.
Sterling, Virginia

Capital Books, Inc.
P.O. Box 605
Herndon, Virginia 20172-0605

Book design and composition by Susan Mark
Coghill Composition Company
Richmond, Virginia

ISBN 10: 1-933102-19-5 (alk. paper)
ISBN 13: 978-1-933102-19-1

**Library of Congress Cataloging-in-Publication Data**

Kocsis, Margaret.
    Savvy eating for the whole family : whole foods, whole family, whole life/
Margaret Kocsis.—1st ed.
        p.   cm.—(Capital's savvy series)
    Includes bibliographical references and index.
    ISBN-13: 978-1-933102-19-1 (pbk. : alk. paper)
    ISBN-10: 1-933102-19-5 (pbk. : alk. paper)
    1. Nutrition.   2. Cookery.   I. Title.   II. Series.
    RA784.K547 2006
    641.5'63—dc22

                                      2005033958

Printed in the United States of America on acid-free paper that meets the American National Standards Institute Z39-48 Standard.

First Edition

10   9   8   7   6   5   4   3   2   1

*To Dad who was the first to prove that Savvy Eating works,
and Mom who inspired me to write in the first place.*

# ACKNOWLEDGMENTS

I would like to thank several people who have helped me bring this book to you. Thanks to Amy Fries and Kathleen Hughes for their editorial skills and support. Thanks to John Dallas, MD, for his valuable advice. Thanks to Stephen Edwards, MD, for his diligence and help. Thanks to Susan Talbert for her encouragement. Special thanks to my family—Paul, John, and Julia—for being testers for all my new recipes, and for their loving support while I was writing and giving seminars.

# CONTENTS

# PREFACE

I have always loved food. I come from a family that associates food with love. Many of us still can't pass a doughnut shop without swerving. Fortunately, my mother taught me early on that you must eat to live rather than live to eat. I've worked hard for many years to balance my love of good food with the desire to be healthy. I studied the scientific research first hand and read the popular books. I experimented with recipes to make them healthier. As a pediatrician, I've had a special interest in nutrition and fitness. Over the past fifteen years, I've treated patients for the whole gamut of nutritional maladies, from obesity and diabetes to anorexia and malnutrition. I've seen first hand what works and doesn't work for my patients and their families. As a result, I came up with a safe, moderate approach to eating well that really works.

Unfortunately, when I tried to convey all that I wanted my patients to know in a short fifteen to thirty minute visit, I became frustrated. I was able to get more across to children and adults alike through the seminars I've taught in schools and in my community. But ultimately, I wanted people to have more than just a handout to take home. Patients would say, "You really have some great suggestions. Can you write them down for me?" I did. This book is especially for my patients and their families.

# CHAPTER 1

# A Fresh Approach to Food

Mrs. Smith sits by herself in the kitchen eating a boiled chicken breast and a tossed salad without dressing while watching the news. The chicken and undressed greens are boring and not very satisfying, and yet she feels virtuous because she is following the latest fad diet. She hopes that this diet will take off that extra twenty pounds she has been trying to lose. Her teenage daughter is eating leftover pizza in her room while on the phone. She has recently become a vegetarian, which by her definition means avoiding animal flesh. It does not in any way imply that one would eat vegetables. The Smith's ten-year-old son is at baseball practice. He will pick up a burger, fries, and a soda with the team on the way home. Mr. Smith is at a business meeting at a fine restaurant. He will come home late, take a few antacids, and watch TV until his heartburn subsides. By then Mrs. Smith is back in the kitchen, looking into the pantry. She feels guilty as she eats a few cookies and chips, but finds herself going back for more.

*Sound familiar?* Mrs. Smith has fallen into the dieting trap while the entire family has forgotten what it's like to enjoy quality food *and* each other's company at the dinner table.

As a pediatrician who has spent the past fifteen years educating patients about nutrition and health, I know how to eat well; yet there was a time when the eating situation in our house was less than ideal. I struggled with cravings for chocolate and sweets. My husband drank soda with meals, frequented fast food eateries at lunch, and rarely ate fruit. My son, the picky eater, objected to all but one vegetable, and my daughter begged for junk food at every meal and snack. There was always the temptation of pizza, fast food, or commercial frozen dinners at the end of a long busy day. In other words, we were average Americans.

## Time to Change

The time has come for a more savvy approach to eating. It's no secret that America's eating is out of control. In my office, we have had to buy larger scales and exam tables to accommodate three-hundred-pound pediatric patients. We have had to learn to recognize and treat children for adult diseases like high blood pressure and type 2 diabetes. Our obese children are suffering from incapacitating orthopedic injuries, depression, and social isolation because of their weight. I see thin teenagers with low energy and thinning hair because they eat a diet of fast food and prepackaged snack foods. As these kids get older, their health problems will only get worse without intervention.

The problem is that our families just don't eat right. Sixty-six percent of American adults and 15 percent of our kids are overweight, and these numbers are growing. Food-influenced diseases like cancer, coronary heart disease, stroke, and diabetes are plaguing our society at unprecedented rates.

In fact, the incidence of these diseases has been steadily increasing over the past century in spite of major advances in disease detection and treatment. More medicines have been developed to combat the diseases resulting from our poor diets, but these medicines frequently have dire side effects, not to mention high price tags. Type 2 diabetes in children was unheard of twenty years ago. Will teenagers who develop type 2 diabetes need dialysis and limb amputations in their thirties? Will our children live shorter lives than their parents? It's quite possible.

## What Can Be Done about America's Eating?

The diet food industry has boomed over the past decade, but to no avail. Quick fix diets cause pain and suffering for the sake of weight loss while often ignoring good nutrition. Dieters are left hungry, frustrated, and no better off than they were before. The return to healthy eating takes a commitment to *lifestyle change* for the whole family, and that is exactly what Americans don't want to hear.

> *The return to healthy eating takes a commitment to lifestyle change for the whole family, and that is exactly what Americans don't want to hear.*

While many people are not happy with the *results* of their poor eating habits, deep down they don't want to change. They're comfortable with their habits and fear that eating better will take too much effort. Some feel that eating out and social affairs will become awkward or embarrassing if they're on a "diet." Others fear they'll be deprived of their favorite comfort foods and the ability to enjoy eating.

Fear not! With a little help, you can actually enjoy eating more! I have developed a philosophy and eating plan based on natural whole foods that brings the enjoyment back to eating. It involves reasonable lifestyle changes that feel good. There are no harsh restrictions or avoidance of food groups. I provide recipes for delicious healthy foods that won't leave you craving junk food. Eating will no longer be a challenge, a chore, or a source of guilt. After reading this book, you too will become a "Savvy Eater." You will

*With a little help, you can actually enjoy eating more! I have developed a philosophy and eating plan based on natural whole foods that brings the enjoyment back to eating.*

- ∾ Learn to eat whole foods that give your body plenty of energy, the ability to fight disease, and the power to heal itself.
- ∾ Decrease your lifetime need for prescription drugs, herbs, and supplements by making savvy food choices.
- ∾ Learn how to avoid foods that harm your body.
- ∾ Avoid cravings through good nutrition.
- ∾ Avoid unwanted weight gain or lose excess weight.
- ∾ Never have to starve yourself to maintain a healthy weight.
- ∾ Learn simple preparations for healthy foods that take no more time to fix than driving out to pick up fast food.
- ∾ Enjoy eating as a family without food battles.
- ∾ Appreciate good food without guilt.

*Sound impossible?* It's not if you take it one step at a time. Changing your eating habits is part of a process. If you asked someone who never exercised to run a mile, they would quickly give up; but if you asked that same person to walk for ten minutes, they could do it.

*Changing your eating habits is part of a process. If you asked someone who never exercised to run a mile, they would quickly give up; but if you asked that same person to walk for ten minutes, they could do it.*

Likewise, I suggest making changes to your diet in ways that are incremental and realistic. My Savvy Eating Plan allows you to change what you can change without dwelling obsessively on the French fries or cake you just couldn't pass up. Savvy Eating will make you feel good, and in some cases, help solve nagging medical problems like heartburn, constipation, and low energy. While I will present evidence-based facts about nutrition and lead you on a path to optimal nutrition, you will choose which advice to incorporate into your life. There is no perfect diet, but every change you make will improve your health.

Savvy Eating not only involves making healthier food choices, but also reducing the stress that many associate with making food choices, preparing food, and getting the family together to eat in peace. Food is meant to be enjoyed and savored, not slaved over and over-contemplated.

# A Developmental Journey

What we eat is a learned behavior. If we had bad eating habits as a child, most likely we have the same bad habits as an adult.

Becoming a healthy eater is a developmental journey. There are developmental milestones that children achieve as they grow. As children, we develop the ability to eat and enjoy new tastes and textures. A six-month-old learns to take solid food from the spoon and swallow it without gagging. A nine-month-old learns to pick up pieces of food and put them in her mouth. Because she's already learned to swallow, she doesn't choke on finger foods. It's necessary for a child to achieve the milestone of swallowing before learning to put foods in her own mouth.

While few children have trouble achieving these basic milestones, many children and adults skipped such milestones as learning to like green vegetables. A child who was rarely offered spinach will probably not like it as a teenager or an adult.

*Children who are not exposed repeatedly and consistently to new tastes learn to favor easy-to-like tastes such as sweets and fats.*

Children who are not exposed repeatedly and consistently to new tastes learn to favor easy-to-like tastes such as sweets and fats.

Even as adults, these people find it a chore to eat more complex foods like vegetables, fish, and whole grains. It doesn't have to be that way. You and your family can learn to enjoy foods that are good for your body.

If you're already fond of a variety of foods, including vegetables and fruits, consider yourself lucky. Savvy Eating will be second nature once you've read the book. If you and your family *don't* enjoy a wide variety of foods, then it will be necessary to go back to the milestone that you missed in your food development and work through it.

When did you learn to prefer fried chicken nuggets to baked chicken? Gummy bears to strawberries? French fries to green beans? As you read about the development of Savvy Eating habits in chapters 3 and 4, you will deal with your own food likes, dislikes, and barriers to good nutrition as you would for a child working through the same issues. When you go back to the milestone that you missed and work through it, the resistance you feel toward change drops, and it becomes easier to eat well.

For instance, you could take one unhealthy food, say doughnuts, and replace them with something healthy that you like, say, whole-grain blueberry muffins. In time, the craving for doughnuts will diminish, and you'll be ready to move on to a new challenge. You may never develop a taste for rutabagas, but acquiring a taste for (and enjoying) beans or broccoli is an easily obtainable goal.

## Healthy Eating Is Easier and Faster than You Think

For many who want to eat well, the difficulty does not lie in their taste preferences, but in their ability to obtain or prepare healthy foods on a consistent basis. You love homemade nutritious dinners, but time is short and Burger King is on the way home. Perhaps you don't know how to prepare seasonal produce in a way that you and your family like, or you're frustrated by complicated labor-intensive recipes. After all, everyone likes commercial mac and cheese and it comes in a box.

*You could take one unhealthy food, say doughnuts, and replace them with something healthy that you like, say, whole-grain blueberry muffins. In time, the craving for doughnuts will diminish, and you'll be ready to move on to a new challenge.*

In the recipe chapters of this book, you will find fast, easy recipes, as well as methods for preparing foods in advance that make it possible to have homemade soups, salads, pastas, and other tasty dishes on the table in less time than it takes to go to McDonald's. Running out for fast food will no longer be a temptation when your pantry is full of good-tasting, healthy food. Once you get the hang of it, preparing healthy whole foods is actually easy.

Veggie pesto pasta cooks in one pot in twenty minutes. Quick to fix and only one pot to clean. Roasted salmon with sweet potatoes and asparagus cooks on aluminum foil faster than the pizza man can deliver. Little to prepare or mix, and clean-up is a snap.

For those who already love to eat healthy foods and are accomplished cooks, the chapters on basic nutrition will be most helpful. You'll learn not to stress over the amount of fat in your diet, why fruits and vegetables are essential and cannot be replaced by supplements, how to improve your health by eating fewer processed foods, and much more.

Most of the changes suggested in these chapters are easy to make. Once you become aware of foods that contain trans fats, for example, it's easy to substitute trans-fat-free brands of snacks, peanut butters, and baked goods for the unhealthy items. Picking up whole grain bread instead of white is easy too. You will discover which fruits and vegetables benefit your body most.

## Think Beyond Cabbage and Tofu

For some with a good knowledge of nutrition, eating has become drudgery. Eating nutritious foods solely because they are good for you is no fun. Trying to force someone else to eat the foods that you know are good for them is pure misery. What's more, it doesn't really work. Food should be savored. When the enjoyment of food dies, nutrition suffers. Consider the story of the Smith family I told at the beginning of this chapter. Don't worry if it sounds all too familiar. In the following chapters, you'll learn how to love healthy foods and enjoy your family's company at the dinner table without stress and worry.

## The Only Real Way to Lose Weight Permanently

For many Americans losing weight is the primary concern. Is it right to put the whole family "on a diet" to help one family member lose weight? Is it right to ostracize the family member trying to lose weight? Should separate meals be prepared for dieting and non-dieting family members? NO. You'll learn to prepare healthy meals for the whole family that everyone will like. You'll also learn about the latest research that enables you to use your own satiety hormones to help you lose weight permanently without hunger.

Before you can make something happen, you must first envision it. You must first believe that it can happen. This chapter began with an all-too-realistic story of eating habits that are devoid of nutrition, as well as pleasure. Try the following exercise. At first it may seemed far-fetched for your family, but with a little imagination and a lot of dedication, you too can make it happen.

*Picture this:* The Smith family is enjoying a satisfying meal of black beans with caramelized onions over aromatic brown rice. The meal is served family-style out on the deck at the end of a fine spring day. Mrs. Smith smiles as her daughter serves herself steamed broccoli (her favorite), and her son chooses the tossed salad with plenty of ranch dressing. For dessert, they have fresh picked strawberries over a vanilla yogurt. They talk about their day: their son's home run and their daughter's math test. Afterwards, Mr. Smith comments on how pleasant the meal has been. They had enjoyed a healthy, inexpensive, and easy-to-fix meal as a family. There was no coercing their formerly picky son to eat his vegetables. Their daughter actually joined them for a meal without criticizing their food choices. They all felt relaxed, satisfied, and energetic.

This can be your reality. The journey starts here.

# CHAPTER 2

# The Shape We're In

## *How Inertia, Uncle Sam, and Clever Advertising Super-sized Americans*

Cornflakes for breakfast, a burger and fries for lunch, pizza for supper, all washed down with a generous amount of Coke. It's no joke! Americans are really eating like this. The modern epidemic of obesity, heart disease, and diabetes is no laughing matter and is directly related to what we eat. While most people eat a little better than the burger, fries, and Coke diet, they're not eating *much* better.

If your diet isn't exemplary, don't be hard on yourself. Eating well today is possibly more difficult than it's ever been. We live in a land of plenty with a variety of nutritious foods available year round that we don't need to grow, harvest, or even prepare for ourselves. However, much of the food we choose to eat is not nutritious, and sometimes it's downright toxic. Why has it become so difficult to choose healthy foods? The reasons are many and have evolved over a long period of time.

Long before the advent of the fast food burger, primitive man hunted and foraged for his food. There were times when there were plenty of berries, nuts, and leafy green things to eat, as well as plentiful game and fish. Man could obtain all of the nutrients he needed from his environment. But throughout history, there were many lean times as well when food was scarce and of low quality. Luckily the human digestive system is somewhat of a garbage can. We can throw just about anything into it and survive for a time. Our ancestors who were able to gorge on food when it was plentiful and store it as fat were the ones who survived. Those with more dainty appetites and less ability to store fat died out in times of famine. The hearty survivors also had a taste preference for sweets and fats. In other words, they liked the foods that allow you to pack in the calories. Genetics definitely play a role in our nation's obesity and chronic-disease epidemic, but they don't tell the whole story.

Anthropologists tell us that our ancestors were not fat even in times of plenty. This is largely due to the fact that primitive people had to chase down the animals they ate and walk much of the day gathering nuts, berries, and other plant foods. We had healthy ancient ancestors who ate diets that consisted almost exclusively of meat. Yet our vegetarian ancestors who ate diets low in protein and fat and high in carbohydrates were healthy too. Even just a few generations ago our ancestors worked on farms or did other physical labor. They walked where they needed to go. Exercise was a necessary part of every day.

That's a far cry from modern man driving to work, swinging through the drive-through for a biscuit, and sitting in front of a computer all day. Energy balance—consuming the same number of calories that you burn through daily activity—is a key factor in preventing obesity and chronic disease. Overeating just one-hundred calories a day (that's about eight ounces of soda) can add up to a weight gain of ten pounds per year. With more overeating or less exercise, the pounds pile on even faster.

Why have we seemingly lost our ancestors' ability to regulate energy balance? Physical inactivity is certainly a key factor, but it's still just a piece of the puzzle. Even our active ancestors may have been a bit more portly if they'd found sweetened sodas, white bread, and French fries hanging on trees.

# Processed Foods:
## Convenience at the Price of Health

Around the turn of the twentieth century, modern technology brought many new foods that do not exist in nature into the human diet. Refined grains such as white wheat flour that had been stripped of its nutrient-containing outer layers and central core became widely available and used. While the refining process did have the advantage of making the grain less prone to spoilage, most of the grain's nutrition was discarded. As the rough outer layer, the bran, is discarded, so are the fiber, magnesium, and other nutrients. Discarding the core of the grain, the germ, throws away many important vitamins like vitamin E, as well as healthy fats.

Fiber and fat take a long time to digest, making you feel satisfied for longer periods of time. Foods like refined flour that are quickly and easily digested and absorbed into the blood stream cause a huge and rapid rise in the body's blood sugar. Foods that cause the body to have these surges in blood sugar are said to have a high glycemic index (GI). Whole-grain, less-refined foods do not cause dramatic surges in blood sugar levels and are said to have a low glycemic index. Diets consisting of primarily high glycemic index foods have been strongly linked to coronary heart disease, type 2 diabetes, and obesity.

---

*Savvy Eating Exercise*

If you haven't experienced the difference that the glycemic index makes, it's worthwhile to self-experiment. Eat a bowl of cornflakes with milk one morning and write down how you feel hourly until 1 p.m. Also record what you ate for lunch and when. The next day have a bowl of old-fashioned oats (prepared in the microwave with a similar amount of milk). Record how you feel hourly until 1 p.m. Again record what you ate for lunch and when. Compare your own satisfaction, as well as how much you ate for lunch.

---

When a high glycemic index food is consumed causing a dramatic rise in blood sugar, the body's natural response is to produce a lot of insulin to help the body process the sugar load. The insulin causes the blood-sugar level to drop, sometimes too far. As the blood sugar drops too low, you feel hungry again. Eating more high GI foods to satisfy your hunger causes another spike in your blood sugar. And thus the roller coaster ride begins. Eating high GI foods causes you to eat more because you feel hungry sooner, even though your body may not yet need to refuel. Low GI foods like unrefined grains, milk, or beans cause the blood sugar to rise slowly. This causes less insulin to be produced and therefore you experience a gradual decline in blood sugar. That's why eating a highly refined cereal like cornflakes leaves you hungry and grouchy by ten thirty, but a bowl of old-fashioned oatmeal with the same number of calories fills you up until noon.

Unfortunately, the study of glycemic index is still in its infancy. You won't find the glycemic index listed on the nutrition panel of your cereal box just yet. Nor is it always evident which foods are refined from looking at the label. "Wheat flour," for example, usually means highly refined white flour, not whole-grain flour. Even "whole wheat flour" can be finely ground and highly processed and therefore yield a bread with a relatively high glycemic index. When grains, even whole grains, are finely ground, they lose some of their ability to slow down digestion and can produce a sharp rise in blood sugar like their white-flour counterparts.

While it's not necessary to eat breads and cereals with the texture of tree bark, we do know that those who eat natural, minimally processed, whole-grain foods feel less hungry, consume less food, and weigh less than those who eat refined grains. Sadly, Americans fell in love with the light and fluffy breads and cakes that could be made with refined flours, and white flour replaced whole-grain flour as a national staple.

# Trans Fats

The plot further thickens with the development of partially hydrogenated oils. Partially hydrogenated oils were created in a chemistry laboratory by bubbling hydrogen gas through heated vegetable oils in the presence of metal particles. This caused a chemical reaction that converted the liquid oil to a solid. These chemically altered oils are called trans fats and have been shown to raise your LDL (the "bad" cholesterol) and lower your HDL (the "good" heart-protective cholesterol), as well as increase your risk of irregular heart beats causing sudden death. Trans fats have proven to be even more harmful than saturated fats. The chemists who developed these fats had no idea what effects they would have on the human body, and trans fats were never tested before they were used in food products. Trans fats became very popular with the food industry because solid fats were easier to transport, and they spoiled more slowly than natural oils. Thus, trans fats became incorporated into most commercial baked goods, including breads, cakes, cookies, and crackers. Trans fats are also widely used for frying chips, French fries, chicken, and other American favorites. Trans fats are so integrally incorporated into our nation's food supply that the food industry is having trouble taking them out of foods now that we know trans fats are dangerous.

The development of partially hydrogenated oils and refined flour, as well as the use of food preservatives, caused the nation's diet to take a further turn for the worse. Cakes, crackers, and white breads that would previously get stale in a day or two could now be packaged in plastic and eaten days or weeks later. These unhealthy foods became not only available but also convenient and inexpensive.

Old-fashioned convenience foods like apples, grapes, and carrots became somewhat frumpy and obsolete compared with snack cakes and chips in neat individual plastic packs. Tasty treats that were previously reserved for special occasions became commonplace, if not expected, in the lunch box of every American child. These nutritionally void snacks frequently replaced nutritious whole grains, proteins, fruits, and vegetables.

As Americans developed a preference for the prepackaged convenience foods over traditional foods, much was lost in the art of food preparation. By the 1950s, convenience foods were the rage. Preparing whole-grain pancakes from scratch was considered a messy waste of time when you could make fluffy white pancakes in a jiffy from a handy refined-flour mix. Just add water, the partially hydrogenated oil is already in the mix! Why serve fresh fruit when you can wow your family with a fruit-flavored gelatin mold? Why bother simmering vegetable soup all afternoon when boiling water can be poured over instant vegetable-flavored soup mix? Who needs actual vegetables when you can have salt-enhanced vegetable flavors? Cooking natural foods from scratch was out of fashion. Fruit, vegetable, and whole-grain food consumption plummeted and type 2 diabetes, heart disease, and obesity skyrocketed.

## Mama Was Right: "Eat Your Vegetables"

Studies show that most modern Americans eat fewer than three vegetables and fruits a day. Fruits and vegetables are our most important source of vital nutrients like vitamins, minerals, and phytochemicals. For most of us, the taste for fruits and especially vegetables is not necessarily love at first sight or first taste for that matter. While most people like the sweet taste of fruits, many don't like fruits' inconsistent texture. Vegetables on the other hand are largely an acquired taste.

> *Fruit, vegetable, and whole-grain food consumption plummeted and type 2 diabetes, heart disease, and obesity sky-rocketed.*

Infants trying bitter or strong-tasting vegetables for the first several times usually reject them. Only after the taste becomes familiar do they eat them by choice. If new foods are not repeatedly introduced to infants, they do not develop the taste for them, making it harder for them to accept them in adulthood. Likewise, adults who do not routinely eat vegetables often lose their taste for them.

When it's easier to satisfy your hunger with a delicious, convenient, although unhealthy snack food, chances are that's what you will do. Preparing and eating fruits and vegetables does take more time than eating a prepared processed food. Unfortunately there is no substitute for eating whole fruits and vegetables. Although modern scientists have isolated many of the vitamins, minerals, and phytochemicals in fruits and vegetables and put them in pill form or added them back into nutrient-depleted refined foods, their effect on the body is not the same as eating the whole food.

> *If new foods are not repeatedly introduced to infants, they do not develop the taste for them, making it harder for them to accept them in adulthood. Likewise, adults who do not routinely eat vegetables often lose their taste for them.*

It's become evident from studies on cancer prevention that the nutrients in fruits and vegetables somehow work in concert to produce their beneficial effects. In other words, the isolated nutrients found in fruits and vegetables don't have the same effect on the body as the intact food. Also, science has not progressed to the point that we know all the nutrients we need to stay healthy. What's more, we don't know the ideal proportions of these nutrients. True vitamin deficiency is rare in the U.S. because many of the known beneficial vitamins and minerals are added into refined foods like cereals and flours. But the vast array of lesser known or unknown phytochemicals that aid in immune function, prevent cancers, and perform other functions in the body are missing or deficient in those who don't eat plenty of fruits and vegetables. Americans should have taken their mothers' advice when they said, "Eat your vegetables!" Our mothers were right.

*There is no substitute for eating whole fruits and vegetables. Although modern scientists have isolated many of the vitamins, minerals and phytochemicals in fruits and vegetables and put them in pill form or added them back into nutrient-depleted refined foods, their effect on the body is not the same as eating the whole food.*

## Misleading Advice on Fats

Unfortunately, Americans didn't listen to their mother's good advice but did accept some bad advice from the government. After studies linked diets high in saturated fat (the type of fat found in meat and full-fat dairy products) with heart disease, the government prepared a policy statement recommending that Americans should eat less red meat. This would have been good advice. But thanks to lobbyists for the meat industry, those recommendations were altered to read "choose a diet low in fat." That's not such good advice.

Diets with moderate amounts of healthy fats like those found in nuts, fish, fruits (like olives and avocados), and grains are beneficial. Decreasing the amount of these beneficial oils in the diet has negative effects on heart health, as well as overall satiety.

*Americans put on weight even faster snacking on low-fat foods than they did eating the often tastier, more satisfying full-fat versions.*

Regrettably, America embraced the low-fat movement wholeheartedly. The food industry went wild marketing low-fat processed foods. The low-fat versions of the foods that flooded the market often contained more sugar and similar amounts of calories to their full-fat counterparts. Sugary refined foods with little fat or fiber are quickly digested leaving you soon hungering for more. Because these foods are low-fat rather than low-calorie, Americans put on weight even faster snacking on low-fat foods than they did eating the often tastier, more satisfying full-fat versions.

## The Super-size Habit

Meanwhile, the food industry seized on Americans' tendency toward overindulgence by marketing larger- and larger-sized packages of foods.

Fast-food companies are particularly guilty of this tactic. In the 1950s, an average fast-food serving of French fries weighed about two ounces and had about two-hundred calories. That's a fairly reasonable indulgence for an active person. By the 1980s, a serving was about four ounces. Now in 2006, a fast-food combo comes with about six ounces of fries and over six-hundred empty calories.

I remember my grandmother opening a twelve-ounce Pepsi-Cola and parceling out a Dixie Cup full to each of us. It was a special treat. She even had a specially designed stopper to keep the remainder of that twelve-ounce bottle fresh until she had the opportunity to finish it. Now fast-food restaurants serve super-sized thirty-two-ounce sodas, often with refills. (Water, it seems, still comes in a small cup.) Cookies, muffins, bagels, and bags of chips have all become grotesquely huge. Modern portion size is way out of proportion to our energy needs, and studies show that people automatically eat more when presented with a larger portion.

Fast foods, TV dinners, and prepackaged snacks have helped move family dinners from the table to the couch in front of the TV. Studies show that people eat more when watching TV than they do sitting at the dinner table. We also miss out on important social interactions that have been shown to decrease stress, increase food satisfaction, and help prevent juvenile delinquency.

*Studies show that people eat more when watching TV than they do sitting at the dinner table.*

Today, the American diet is full of trans fat and refined grains and sugars in super-sized portions, while it's seriously deficient in fiber, vitamins, minerals, antioxidants, and healthy oils. It took a long time for the American diet to evolve into its current state of disrepair, so fixing our diet woes can take some time and effort. Recommendations that would be rather straight-forward and easy-to-follow in another era are complex today because too many choices are available.

The average person needs guidance to become a Savvy Eater. Read on and you will find a guide for children and adults alike who need help developing a taste for healthier foods, a concise explanation of the reasoning and evidence behind the above dietary guidelines, and methods for incorporating Savvy Eating as painlessly as possible into your lifestyle.

## Summary

The best place to start developing Savvy Eating habits is to make the changes that will have the largest impact on your health. The most important guidelines can be boiled down to the following:

1. Eat a variety of fruits and vegetables (at least five to nine servings a day).
2. Choose minimally processed whole grains over refined grains
   and sugars.
3. Substitute healthy fats for saturated and trans fats.
4. Choose healthy protein sources like fish, lean chicken, beans,
   and nuts, and eat plenty of protein throughout the day.
5. Develop a sense of portion size that enables you to enjoy a
   variety of foods while maintaining a stable healthy weight.

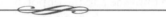

# CHAPTER 3

# The Development of Savvy Eating

## *Babies and Toddlers*

Early childhood is the time when our eating habits and food preferences are developed. Healthy childhood eating habits, such as drinking milk rather than soda, eating vegetables daily, and ending a meal when satisfied not full, are likely to carry over into healthy adult eating practices. Unhealthy practices such as drinking sweet beverages, frequenting fast-food restaurants, and overeating are likely to persist into adulthood too. Patterns established in childhood—for better or for worse—are difficult to change.

If you and your family members developed healthy eating habits as children, consider yourself lucky. If you didn't, it's not too late to change. First, recall your own childhood habits. Did you like a variety of vegetables, or were you a picky eater? Were you bold and adventurous with new food, or did you stick to comfort foods like macaroni and cheese? Did your parents indulge your sweet tooth, or were they restrictive with sodas and sweets? Did you eat at the family table or in front of the TV?

The development of food preferences follows a pattern throughout childhood. In this chapter I'll discuss the development of healthy eating habits. When you come to a milestone that you have not yet mastered, work through it as you would for a child. Give yourself time. Thirty years of eating fast food is not going to give way to homemade vegetarian dinners overnight. Like infants, you must develop new tastes over time. Also, don't force family members to eat things they don't want. Instead, consistently provide them with healthy food choices appropriate for their developmental level. They too will take time to adjust their palate.

> *Thirty years of eating fast food is not going to give way to homemade vegetarian dinners overnight. Like infants, you must develop new tastes over time.*

## How to Help Your Child Develop Good Lifelong Eating Habits

Studies show that the single most important thing you can do to promote healthy eating habits in your child is to model healthy eating habits your-self. When children see their parents eating vegeta-bles, resisting seconds, and eating well, they are likely, in time, to do the same. When children see their parents drinking sweetened beverages, eating until they are full, and snacking on chips while watching TV, that is what they will do too. Ad-monishing your child for his eating choices while making poor choices yourself is counterproduc-tive. "Do what I say, not as I do" doesn't go over well with kids.

> *Studies show that the single most important thing you can do to promote healthy eating habits in your child is to model healthy eating habits yourself.*

## Savvy Eating Starts with Baby Food

*What can I do to instill healthy eating habits from birth?* A full discussion of infant feeding is beyond the scope of this book, but I will discuss a few of the key milestones in the development of food preferences and eating habits. If some of these milestones are missed, don't despair, your child is not destined for poor eating habits. But following these suggestions as your child grows will make it easier for him to adopt good eating habits.

### BREASTFEED

The most important thing you can do for your newborn, if at all possible, is to breastfeed for at least twelve months. Breastfed infants are healthier and are less likely to become overweight adults.

### RELAX

Show your child the right attitude toward food—food is to be enjoyed and eaten only until hunger is satisfied. Infants start to eat solid foods at four to six months of age. During this stage, babies get most of their nutrition from breast milk or formula, so parents can relax and have a "take it or leave it" approach to solid foods. Remember, it's your job to start offering solids, not to make sure that they're eaten.

By six months, most infants are ready to be offered a new fruit, veg-etable, or infant cereal every five to seven days. They will learn to like most of the foods to which they're exposed. Some foods babies will like from the first bite, and others they will like only after trying them ten to twenty times. *Yes, ten to twenty times.* Many parents assume that a child does not like a food because he refuses it three or four times. While you must accept that some foods will never be liked, it's wise to offer green beans over and over again even if they end up on the bib. Many children will refuse all or most new foods the first few times they're offered.

### CULTIVATE A PLAYFUL ATTITUDE

Having a playful attitude and a smile on your face during feedings is more important than what your child eats from the spoon at this age. Your pediatrician will be following your child closely to make

*Some foods babies will like from the first bite, and others they will like only after trying them ten to twenty times. Yes, ten to twenty times. Many parents assume that a child does not like a food because he refuses it three or four times. While you must accept that some foods will never be liked, it's wise to offer green beans over and over again even if they end up on the bib.*

---

## Savvy Eating Tips for Adult Picky Eaters

If there is an adult or older child in your family who never learned to like a variety of tastes and textures, it's probably because he was a cautious eater. Chances are he required more than just a few exposures to foods to learn to like them, and understandably, caregivers became frustrated and gave up offering new foods before he grew to accept them.

New healthy foods should be consistently provided for picky adults as well as children. For older kids and adults who won't eat vegetables, it's a good idea to figure out what they don't like about them. Is it the texture, the look, or the taste?

- If it's the texture, try making smooth-textured cream of broccoli soup or try shredding salads into uniform little bits.
- If it's the look, try sprinkling the offending food with cheese or dipping in dressing or ketchup.
- If it's the taste, just like with infants, the first step toward acceptance is tolerating the new food on the plate. He will eventually progress to trying a small bite, then, after many more exposures, a serving; perhaps he'll even learn to like the new food. Remember, it's OK to offer the food and even to ask that an older child or adult try it, but do not cajole, bribe, or force him to eat.

sure he is growing well and getting good nutrition. He will recommend a vitamin or iron supplement if necessary. So relax and enjoy feedings for what they are: messy food exploration.

Provide a good example by being happy and adventurous with food, while refraining from pushing food once your child is satisfied. When he turns his head, closes his lips, and looks away from the food, chances are he is through. That means leaving that little bit of sweet potatoes in the jar rather than trying to make him finish them.

*Provide a good example by being happy and adventurous with food, while refraining from pushing food once your child is satisfied.*

Unfortunately, many children start to lose their self-regulatory abilities at an early age. Bottle fed infants are often encouraged to finish an arbitrary amount of formula in their bottles, even if they're satisfied. Some babies are encouraged to eat a measured amount of cereal whether they're hungry or not. These babies learn to eat until stuffed. This may be part of the reason that breastfed babies are less likely than bottle fed babies to be overweight children and adults. Follow your baby's cues. Stop feeding when he loses interest.

Meal times are an important social time spent with the whole family. Make sure you sit with your child at meals so he can see you enjoying a variety of foods. Your child will learn to sit peacefully in his chair and enjoy his food if you are sitting too. Kids who fight the high chair usually have family members that don't sit with them.

### At the Right Time, Branch Out with Caution

By the time your child is nine-months-old, he's ready to branch out and try new textures and finger foods. He'll take pride in picking up foods and feeding himself and may want less help from you. This is the right time to start slowly and cautiously introducing your child to mashed table foods. Set the food out in bowls on the table. Pass the bowls to older family members and let them serve themselves. Let toddlers point to foods they would like to try. Offer infants table foods in turn, but let your child decide how much of, or even if he is going to try a food. Children are more likely to accept a new food if trying it in the first place is their own idea.

Learning to like mashed table food is a key developmental milestone. If your baby learns to eat what you're eating, you won't be stuck preparing separate meals for the adults and the kids for the next ten years. Granted, some adult foods are inappropriate for young children, especially if they're very spicy or difficult to chew. That's when you're stuck modifying the meal or making two meals. However, many of the soups, pasta dishes, and rice dishes in this book are ideal for little ones as well as adults. As long as you offer them to your children on a regular basis, healthy foods will become comfort foods and staples in your child's diet.

A child that refuses solids at nine months is unusual and should be brought to your pediatrician's attention. It's more common for them to be putting everything in their mouths. At this time your job broadens from being a tour guide in food adventures to being a gatekeeper and protector.

The main concerns at this age are protecting your child from potential choking hazards, potential allergens, and unhealthy yet attractive convenience foods.

- ∞ To avoid choking, infants and toddlers need to be offered only small pieces of mashed foods or foods that can easily dissolve in the mouth with minimal chewing.
- ∞ Because of the potential for allergic reactions, infants should never have whole eggs, seafood, nuts or nut butters, or dairy products like milk, cheese, and yogurt before twelve months of age. After a year, these foods can gradually be added to his diet one at a time. It's a good idea to wait until three years of age to give nuts or nut butters because they're choking hazards. Also, children with early exposure to nuts are more likely to develop peanut allergy. Allergy to peanuts and nuts tends to be life long and is often more severe than other allergies, therefore well worth avoiding.
- ∞ Avoid honey until after a year of age to prevent botulism, a potentially deadly condition caused by bacterial spores that can be found in honey.

### FINGER FOODS AND SNACKS

Usually the biggest problem at this age is limiting your child to foods that are healthy. Because they can pick up, chew, and swallow graham crackers, cookies, and goldfish crackers, and it gives them great pleasure to do so, parents often succumb to both peer pressure and to their child's insistence on eating these fun foods. These processed unhealthy foods have no place in an infant's diet. The longer you can avoid introducing him to these foods, the better. Consider also that most cookies and crackers contain dairy products (which they shouldn't have until a year), refined sugar, refined white flour, and trans fats.

It's tempting to offer kids unhealthy yet convenient snack foods because they are too young for many healthy snacks like raw vegetables, hard fruits, and nuts. Fortunately, kids love snacks like toasted oat cereal (Cheerios), bits of toasted whole-grain bread, cooked whole-grain pasta,

> *Savvy Eating Tips:*
> *Food Should Be Eaten While Seated to Avoid Choking*
>
> Wandering around while eating snacks is dangerous and encourages your child to graze rather than sit with the family for meals and snacks. Children learn social skills and good eating habits from watching adults at the table. If you put a child in a high chair or booster chair every time he eats (including snacks), you won't have as hard a time keeping him in the high chair for meals. You'll also spend less time cleaning up mashed Cheerios and juice spots in other rooms of your house.

soft fruit, and even chopped cooked veggies. Don't worry about offering a huge variety of finger foods for snacks. Snacks can be basic as kids get a great deal of variety learning to eat chopped-up table foods at mealtimes.

Remember that unless toddlers are taught that snacks usually come in little plastic packages, they're content to eat healthy foods for snacks as well as meals.

Next time you see a toddler wandering around grazing on snack food, consider that the average baggie-full of goldfish crackers often has about 150 calories. The total energy needs of an average one year old is often only around 1000 calories a day. That package of junk food may be an eighth of that child's daily calorie requirement. No wonder he's not hungry for supper.

# Finicky Toddlers

Sometime between a year and two years, ravenous little babies become finicky toddlers. They are growing more slowly and eat much less food than they did in previous months. Parents are often frustrated because their toddler just seems to play with food, not really eat it. They often consume only a few mouthfuls at a meal, but somehow manage to paint the whole kitchen with peas and carrots. They'll put a new food in their mouth only to take it back out again. This is their way of learning about new foods. Knowing that this behavior is normal can help you feel less stressed about your child's eating habits.

This is the age when it's difficult and yet very important to stand firm. Continue to offer healthy foods to your child, even if very little is being eaten. Don't give in and buy junk food just so he'll eat. If the healthy food is there when he finally gets hungry, then that's what he'll eat. Your child will develop taste preferences based on what he is exposed to the most often. If he eats fruits, vegetables, and whole grains most often, then that's what he'll like. If he's given chicken nuggets or pizza every time he balks at a meal, then that's what he'll prefer.

*Your child will develop taste preferences based on what he is exposed to the most often. If he eats fruits, vegetables, and whole grains most often, then that's what he'll like. If he's given chicken nuggets or pizza every time he balks at a meal, then that's what he'll prefer.*

Most kids, and especially cautious kids (a.k.a. picky eaters), want foods with predictable textures. That's part of the reason so many kids get into a rut eating chicken nuggets, French fries, macaroni and cheese, and peanut butter sandwiches. They know exactly what to expect: no unpredictable lumps, stringy things, or intense flavors. These foods are easy to like. Cautious kids don't like most foods at first bite, especially if the food falls into the "unpredictable" category. Parents often become frustrated with food refusal and give up offering healthy foods. However, if cautious kids are repeatedly exposed to healthy foods like carrot soup, bean burritos, and oatmeal, they'll become favorite comfort foods rather than unhealthy typical American fare.

*If cautious kids are repeatedly exposed to healthy foods like carrot soup, bean burritos, and oatmeal, they'll become favorite comfort foods rather than unhealthy typical American fare.*

The toddler years into the preschool years are the time to make sure that you don't enter into food battles. Accept that your child will be picky or hardly eat at times, and don't worry about it as long as your child's pediatrician says that your child is growing normally. Resist the temptation to give your child junk food because he whines for it. Setting the ground rules now will save you a lot of trouble later.

## Let the Portion Fit the Child

If your hungry child often balks when served a plate with two vegetables, meat, fruit, and pasta, even if he likes the food, he's probably overwhelmed. Make sure you're not offering unreasonable portions. (Most fruits and vegetable servings are about one tablespoon per year of age up to age eight). Small children can easily be overwhelmed when faced with too many choices or by a large amount of food on their plate. Try serving the meal family style, with all the dishes of food on the table. Ask a young child which foods he wants, spoon a small serving onto his plate, and ask if that's enough. You can offer additional foods once the first round is eaten.

*Accept that your child will be picky or hardly eat at times, and don't worry about it as long as your child's pediatrician says that your child is growing normally.*

## DON'T RESORT TO FORCE

*My child often refuses food or just picks at it. How do I get my child to eat?* Children are often not hungry when we offer food, and other times they stubbornly refuse certain foods even when they are hungry. Never force your child to eat if he's not hungry. Imagine how stressful it would be to be forced to eat when you are full. Being stuffed is a miserable feeling.

Imagine having someone forcing you to eat an unfamiliar food. A good example would be the fabled Bertie Bott's Every Flavor Beans from *Harry Potter*. They come in *every* flavor. Will it be toffee flavor or ear wax? Strawberry or spinach? Will you be able to spit it out if you don't like it? If you're a naturally daring person, you might not mind risking a bad taste. However, if you're a cautious eater, having to try a new food or a food that was a previous bad experience can be very stressful.

Parental pressure to eat does account for a modest (about 15 percent) change in a child's eating behavior, but that change doesn't have a significant impact on a child's diet. It does, however, have the potential for negative side effects. Forcing a child to eat a new, unwanted, or disliked food usually backfires. The forced food becomes a hated food to be avoided at all costs. In extreme situations, when foods are forced on a child on a regular basis, the child becomes defensive when any food is offered.

> *Children who are forced to eat develop fears of new foods and anxiety associated with eating that can possibly lead to eating disorders.*

Children who are forced to eat develop fears of new foods and anxiety associated with eating that can possibly lead to eating disorders. The child refuses to eat except for a very limited number of foods, and mealtimes become unpleasant battles.

## *Summary*

To develop Savvy Eating habits in infants and toddlers, parents should provide their children with safe and healthy foods and approach mealtimes with an easy-going attitude.

1. Be a good example. Kids model their eating behavior after their parents. You may need to work through developmental issues with your own eating habits.

2. Keep safety in mind. Make sure the foods you serve are appropriate for your child's age and development and make sure that everyone sits to eat.

3. Have a relaxed attitude toward food. It's not your job to make a family member eat nutritious food. Your job is to provide healthy foods on a regular basis.

4. Make snacks as healthy as meals. They're a significant part of your family's diet.

# CHAPTER 4

# The Development of Savvy Eating

## *Preschool and School-Age Children*

As your child transitions from being a toddler to a preschooler, the social aspects of eating take center stage. It's time to set the ground rules for good eating.

## Establishing Good Lifetime Eating Habits and Avoiding Food Wars

### SET THE TIME, PLACE, AND THE TABLE

It's important to have set times for meals and snacks. Unpredictable eating habits and allowing kids (or adults) to graze make it more difficult to self-regulate food intake. This usually leads to overeating. Letting kids over a year of age eat on demand encourages consumption of unhealthy convenience foods, especially if they're allowed to eat anywhere other than the table. Even if your child is willing to eat leftover spaghetti and salad for snack, you might find yourself offering a bag of chips instead if they're used to eating snacks on the sofa. Predictable meal and snack times, as well as eating at the table, make healthy eating easier in the long run.

### TURN OFF THE TV AND EAT AT THE FAMILY TABLE

Eating meals as a family at the table at least once a day is essential to the development of healthy eating habits. Children learn important skills watching their parents at the table. They learn to sit while eating, develop table manners, and over time, acquire tastes for new foods. Kids learn by example. Model behaviors you would like them to have. Even if your own habits don't set the perfect example, sharing meals together helps strengthen family bonds. Eating at the family table gives family members a chance to com-

*Eating meals as a family at the table at least once a day is essential to the development of healthy eating habits.*

## Savvy Eating Tips: The Family Table

- Encourage young children to set the table. Ask them to put out the plates, napkins, and silverware. Toddlers will take pride in having a job to do. Older children who were taught to do this at an early age will set the table as a matter of course without grumbling.
- Sit at the table and take a moment to give thanks. No matter what your religious beliefs, expressing gratitude is a healthy behavior.
- Turn off the TV and don't allow reading or toys at the table during the meal. (That includes the newspaper!) If possible, do not answer the phone.
- Discuss the day's events and what you're looking forward to. Avoid controversial topics.
- Put food on the table in bowls with serving spoons and allow everyone to serve their own plate. Start this by age three.
- Everyone should remain seated during the meal, but can be excused when they're finished.
- Everyone (above the age of three) should take their own plate to the kitchen after the meal. Older children should have more responsibility.
- Make family meals a priority. Adjust schedules whenever possible to allow the family to eat together daily, even if its breakfast.

municate face to face. This aspect of eating at the family table has been shown to help prevent juvenile delinquency.

If the older children and adults in your family eat in front of the TV instead of at the family table, it's time to break that habit.

It's important to learn how to enjoy food without distraction for a variety of reasons. When we learn to be mindful about what we're putting in our mouths, we tend to make better choices. Kids who are distracted by things like TV eat more than they would if they were sitting at the table. To make matters worse, the foods Americans typically eat in front of the TV are less healthy than those eaten at meals. Also, certain television shows (usually the ones aimed at children) are loaded with commercials that glamorize junk food. Why tempt them? Turn off the TV for snacks and meals and help your kids avoid shows that are heavy on junk food ads.

Remember, studies show that when people eat in front of the TV they

- ∾ Eat more food and eat faster
- ∾ Feel less satisfied
- ∾ Eat fewer healthy foods and more junk food
- ∾ Feel more isolated

## A HEALTHY VIEW ON TEMPTATION

As children start preschool and grade school, they're exposed to a lot of eating habits that are out of your control. Even if you pack all of your child's meals and snacks, she'll notice what other kids are eating, and Pandora's Box is opened. It's difficult for her to see why she should eat vegetables when she sees her friends eating salty fish-shaped crackers, snack-cakes with sprinkles, and brightly colored sugar water in a pouch. Thanks to effective marketing, these types of foods are irresistible to most kids. Many parents are determined not to expose their children to these unhealthy snacks, and that's a good approach for the first year or so of life. But unless your children don't go to school and never play with other kids, you cannot shelter them from knowing about these foods for long.

The most reasonable approach to keeping these unhealthy foods from tempting your children is to avoid keeping them in the house, but not re-stricting your child from having a reasonable serving when they attend a party or go to a friend's house. If you restrict your child from eating the "forbidden foods" even at parties, your child will usually react by desiring the forbidden item even more. Studies show that when a restricted child is away from his parent at school or at a party where she has access to the "forbidden food," she will often gorge herself on that food until she is stuffed.

## WHEN DESSERTS AND SNACKS LEAVE NO ROOM FOR VEGGIES

*My child is always "too full" for vegetables, but ready to eat dessert.* Choosing to eat healthy foods can be problematic for children. Respect your child's ability to know when she's satisfied and don't push her to clean her plate if she's full. However, if your child is pushing away from the table before she's satisfied in hopes of filling up on ice cream and cook-ies, refrigerate her leftovers and serve them as her next snack or meal. For food safety reasons, be sure that food has not been out for more than an hour if you plan to re-serve it.

If your child suddenly becomes hungry again when dessert or another desirable food becomes available, stand your ground and serve her her leftover meal. If she is still hungry after eating her meal, then offer the dessert or snack. (If she's full after finishing her meal, reassure her that the dessert or desired food will be available to her at another time when she's hungry.) If this strategy is used regularly, it helps avoid the common scenario of being too full for broccoli but hungry for cake.

Food battles with children can be exasperating. It's imperative that you remain calm when dealing with these situations. Knowing that limit testing, food refusal, and strange or picky eating habits are all normal childhood behaviors can help defuse the frustration and anger you may feel when you and your children clash wills over food issues. It pays to have a plan: Accept the food refusal, but don't offer other foods to bribe her to eat. Calmly execute your plan: remove the plate from the table and refrigerate it for snack time. Eventually your child will catch on.

*Knowing that limit testing, food refusal, and strange or picky eating habits are all normal childhood behaviors can help defuse the frustration and anger you may feel when you and your children clash wills over food issues.*

*I have tried accepting food refusal and re-serving leftovers. My child just won't eat anything but chicken nuggets!* You may not have let the child know that you're serious about eating healthy foods. If you appease the child by offering a favorite food when she refuses other foods, *even occasionally*, you've undermined your efforts to help her learn to like new foods. You need to demonstrate that

---

### Savvy Eating Tips: Dessert Dilemmas

Don't require your child to finish his meal in order to get dessert. If pining for dessert becomes a problem, consider serving a small dessert with the meal and letting your child eat it when she wants, with the understanding that the portion she has received is all there is.

If you choose to serve dessert on a regular basis, make desserts healthy some of the time. Kids like strawberry smoothies, fresh fruit, popsicles made from 100 percent fruit juice, chocolate milk, and bananas with chocolate syrup as much as other more decadent desserts. (See the chapter on desserts for more kid-friendly dessert ideas.) Remember desserts don't have to be sweets. Popcorn, nuts, or even dried apricots and dates are great treats at the end of a meal.

Keep in mind that every food you put on the table need not be a favorite with your child even if it's dessert. Serving "grown up" desserts like dried fruit and nuts or fruit and cheese help teach your child that treats are not always sweets or unhealthy foods. Conversely, they'll also learn that dessert is not always the best part of the meal.

when she says she is not hungry, you will let her leave the table and re-frigerate her food until she is hungry. Ask her to sit with the family at the table for a few minutes and tell you about her day. She may decide she's hungry after all. If not, let her leave the table. Don't offer milk, cereal, or juice or any other food when she finally gets hungry. Offer her the saved meal when it's time for the next meal or snack. Don't offer food at any time other than set meal and snack times. The average preschool child must see you demonstrate this fifteen to twenty times before she'll accept it as the rule. Once the rule is established you just have to be consistent.

If you continue to offer your child nourishing food alternatives, she will not starve to death. Many children have impressive will power and will refuse to eat several meals in a row before try-ing a new or undesired food. Being hungry for a few hours or even overnight is not cruel as long as you have offered her food. It is rare that a child will need to go to bed hungry more than two or three times before understanding that you mean business.

> *The only reason a child will refuse all foods but chicken nuggets or another favorite food, is because an adult is continuing to give that food to the child.*

The *only* reason a child will refuse all foods but chicken nuggets or another favorite food, is be-cause an adult is continuing to give that food to the child. When a child refuses to eat nourishing food, unhealthy foods need to be unavailable, at least until he has learned to accept healthy foods.

## OFFER HEALTHY FOODS ON YOUR CHILD'S TERMS

In all fairness to your child, you should offer at least one familiar and liked food at each meal.

Never feed your child something you would not eat yourself. It's also a good rule of thumb to offer no more than one new food per meal unless your child is very adventurous. When the family is eat-ing spicy, odd textured, or strong-tasting foods, simply offer that food. If she tries it, reward your child with praise, not dessert.

> *In all fairness to your child, you should offer at least one familiar and liked food at each meal.*

- ∾ Don't automatically put new foods on her plate and insist that she eat them. Let her approach a new food at her own pace.
- ∾ Use your judgment. Kids can reasonably be expected to like split pea soup even if it's green, but spicy curry or octopus salad might be expecting too much.
- ∾ Accept that young children are not usually casserole eaters. Most kids like each food to be separate rather than combined in

---

### Savvy Eating Tips: Help Picky Kids Become Healthy Eaters

Some children readily accept new foods, and others will never try new foods without encouragement. If your child falls into the latter category, then try positive reinforcement for trying new foods. Use star (or sticker) charts or small rewards for trying (not finishing) new foods. Avoid using food rewards. Your child may be tempted to stuff herself to get her treat, and this can undermine your child's ability to self-regulate food intake.

If your child doesn't like to eat vegetables, you can use star charts to reward them for eating three vegetables a day. When she gets a certain number of stars, she can see a video, get a small toy, or earn a trip to the park. If your child begs to eat fast food in order to get the kid's meal toy, offer a similar toy or purchase the desired toy from the restaurant as a star chart prize.

Because the star chart is a visual form of praise rather than an immediate food reward, children are not as likely to stuff themselves to get the star.

---

a dish with sauce. They often don't even want their foods touching on the plate. When you prepare a dish with pasta, chicken, vegetables, and sauce, you may need to serve your child the individual components separately and let her dip them in the sauce if she's feeling daring that day.

### Don't Be Sneaky

Including vegetables in your child's diet by stealth can have mixed results. Hard-core picky eaters may accept carrot muffins and pasta dishes with shredded broccoli stalks hidden in them, but your child might resent the sneak factor if he detects the presence of unwanted foods. Be honest. Your best bet is to be persistent in offering healthy foods and making unhealthy foods unavailable.

*Your best bet is to be persistent in offering healthy foods and making unhealthy foods unavailable.*

For those who don't get five to nine servings of fruits and vegetables a day, a daily children's multivitamin is also a good idea.

### Make Food Fun

Make food fun and interesting. Let kids make happy faces or designs with raw veggies, then eat them with dip. Dip apple slices or veggies in peanut butter. A teaspoonful of mini chocolate chips or a sprinkle of powdered sugar can go a long way toward making yogurt, oatmeal, or fresh fruit more enticing without adding a significant number of calories. Try fun pasta shapes: bow ties, twists, and alphabets. Offer healthy drinks like skim milk and water in unusually shaped cups or bottles or with fun straws. Food that looks visually appealing is more likely to be eaten.

Visual appeal can work both ways. Thanks to extensive market research, nothing is more visually appealing to kids than junk food. Junk foods are foods with low nutrient density (LND). In other words, they have very little nutritional value for the amount of calories they contain. An active child who eats healthy foods is very unlikely to become overweight, but a child who eats junk food (LND foods) regularly is very much at risk of being overweight.

## LET YOUR CHILD HELP CHOOSE AND MAKE FOOD

As your child gets older, enlist your child's help in choosing or making food. Let him help make a peanut butter sandwich or toss a salad. Say, "Would you like yogurt or bananas for your snack?" rather than asking an open-ended question like, "What do you want for a snack?" (The answer might be "ice cream"!)

## NOBODY BUT YOUR CHILD KNOWS
## HOW MUCH SHE NEEDS TO EAT

It's important not to force a child to eat a certain amount of food. The amount a child needs to eat varies widely with her energy output for that

---

### Savvy Eating Info: Low Nutrient Density Foods

*What are low nutrient density foods?* Low Nutrient Density Foods (LND foods) have relatively little nutritional value for the amount of calories they contain. Prime examples of LND foods are cookies and other sweets, crackers, pretzels, chips, puffed rice cakes, sweet cereals, sweetened drinks, fried foods (even "veggie" chips), and bread and pasta made with white flour, corn, or white rice.

Those who eat LND foods consume more calories and have more cravings than those who eat nutrient dense foods like fruits, vegetables, low-fat dairy products, and whole grains. Studies show that eating more low nutrient density foods correlates with increased incidence of obesity.

day, her age, and how much she's growing. No adult can accurately gage exactly how much a child needs to eat at a certain meal. Letting a child develop a sense of how much food he needs is pivotal to keeping a child from becoming overweight. Forcing a child to "clean her plate" whether she is full or not undermines her natural ability to regulate her food intake. Members of the Clean Plate Club learn to eat until stuffed out of habit.

### Let Young Children Serve Themselves

Preschool-age kids and older can serve their own plates, and you should let them do this whenever possible. They'll be more adventurous with food and develop a better ability to self-regulate if they're allowed to decide which foods and how much they'll eat. There will be mistakes in judging the amount of food to take as well as spills, but this is all an important part of learning to eat well.

### Don't Over Restrict

Children with too many food restrictions are also more likely to have difficulty regulating their food intake as adults. Restricted children are more likely to develop obesity or an eating disorder as a teen or an adult. It's best to be honest with children and explain why you don't buy unhealthy foods. School-age children are old enough to understand a basic explanation of why you would like them to eat well. Say, "I don't buy chips (or sweet drinks, crackers, or whatever food is being begged for) because they have chemicals (like sugar, trans fats, dyes, and preservatives) in them that harm our bodies and because they can make us feel bad if we eat too many of them." End the conversation there. Do not apologize, bargain, or rationalize.

### Don't Dwell on Food Issues

Don't talk about food choices any more than is absolutely necessary. Dwelling on food is more likely to make a child rebellious or overly concerned with food choices. Continue to offer healthy food choices and praise your child for making healthy choices on her own. (Don't, however, make a big deal about good food choices. Children who love to please can become performers, often eating past the point of satiety in order to get praise and please their parents.) Talk about how healthy foods make us feel good and strong and give us energy to do fun things. Don't comment on foods making you big or fat.

---

### Savvy Eating Tips: Eating Disorders

The exact causes of anorexia nervosa and other eating disorders are not known. Stress, lack of family support and communication, anxiety, depression, and genetics play important roles. It's not known whether overemphasis on food choices, labeling foods as "good" and "bad," or talking about a child's size influences the development of eating disorders. However, building positive family relationships and social skills by eating at the family table, while allowing kids to regulate their food intake by serving themselves may give them some protection against eating disorders.

---

### AVOID THE FAST FOOD HABIT

People who frequent fast food establishments eat fewer vegetables, fruits, and whole grains. They eat more processed foods and more calories. Eating fast foods dramatically increases your chances of becoming obese. Kids who eat a monotonous diet of French fries, cheese burgers, chicken nuggets, and ice cream do not learn to like fruits and vegetables and grow to prefer processed breads to whole grains. If you must go to fast food restaurants, make sure your child eats salads, fruit, and milk at least as often as burgers and fries.

### WATCH THE DRINKS

Teach your child that water is the beverage that quenches thirst. While skim milk and occasionally 100 percent fruit juice are a part of a healthy diet, train your child to reach for water when she's thirsty. Milk and juices are foods that one drinks when hungry. Don't buy sodas, fruit drinks, or

---

### Savvy Eating Tip: The Ideal Kid Food

If you always wondered how your grandmother managed to raise eight healthy children without the help of graham crackers or happy meals, it's because she fed them the ideal kid food, soup. Messy, yes, but homemade soup is loaded with vegetables cooked to softness, little bits of tender meat, and flavorful broth. Kids love it. See my recipes for soups starting on page 159.

sweet tea. They have no place in a child's diet. A twelve-ounce soda has 150 empty calories. Even fast food kid's meals offer milk or water as an option. Set a good example. If your child sees you drinking a sweet beverage, she will inevitably want some. Save sweet drinks for special occasions.

## Concerns for Underweight Children

It is best to respect your child's ability to self-regulate the amount of food she eats. This is especially true for children who are either overweight or failing to thrive. Underweight children respond to food forcing by eating less, not more. As a parent, it's difficult but imperative that you don't stress over every bite that your child does or doesn't put in her mouth.

I've often been to children's parties where the concerned parent of a thin child tries to bargain with her two-year-old, "Eat just two more bites of pizza and you can have some cake," as if those two bites of junk food were somehow going to make her child a bigger, stronger, healthier person. The child is often wandering around rather than seated safely as the furrow-browed parent is trying to poke pizza in her disinterested or outright resistant child's mouth. The child is more interested in normal social activities like playing than eating. The parent is often totally unaware of how absurd her actions appear to others. It's a party. It's time to relax about eating and celebrate.

Children who routinely refuse for their cajoling parents will often eat normally when fed by another caregiver, especially if that person both sits and eats with the child and has a relaxed attitude toward food. So parents need to learn to ease off. The child may not eat much more at first, but once she learns to trust that you will not force her to eat, she'll develop better eating habits and gain weight according to her genetic ability.

## Dealing with Overweight Children

By the same token, it's difficult to back off when your pediatrician has told you your child is overweight. Withholding food from overweight children makes them fear that they'll not get enough to eat. Overweight children tend to eat faster and take larger bites in the presence of a restrictive parent, presumably so they can fill up before food is taken away. They'll also sneak food or binge on food when it becomes available without supervision. As the parent of an overweight child, it's not your responsibility to restrict how much food your child eats. You read correctly. However, it *is* your responsibility to

∾ decide when and where food will be eaten (Preferably at the table, away from the TV, at designated meal and snack times)
∾ provide healthy foods for your child
∾ decrease the availability of low nutrient density foods.

Your child is also at increased risk of obesity if she spends two or more hours a day in front of the TV, computer, or video games. In most cases, an overweight child will lose weight if provided with a healthy diet, restricted to no more than one hour of TV a day, and encouraged to exercise daily. Children and teens need a *minimum* of one hour of vigorous physical activity a day.

*Approximately, 20 percent of overweight young children and 80 percent of overweight adolescents become overweight adults.*

The percentage of overweight children in our country has dramatically increased over the last thirty years. Approximately, 20 percent of overweight young children and 80 percent of overweight adolescents become overweight adults.

Studies show that the most important thing a parent can do to prevent their child from becoming overweight is to model good eating habits themselves.

Having a parent who is overweight is a much stronger predictor of whether a child will grow up to be overweight than a young child's own weight.

*Having a parent who is overweight is a much stronger predictor of whether a child will grow up to be overweight than a young child's own weight.*

While genes certainly contribute to a child's weight, family eating patterns have a huge influence. Children who are given large or adult-sized portions are more likely to consume more calories than when they are served child-sized portions or allowed to serve themselves. Serving young children on child-sized plates helps limit portion size. Keep in mind that fast-food kids' meals often contain adult-sized portions of chicken nuggets, cheeseburgers, and fries with unlimited refills on sweet drinks. Children who eat at fast-food establishments eat significantly more calories than when they eat at home. If you or your child is overweight, avoiding fast-food restaurants is imperative.

There are six specific things that you can do to help prevent your child from becoming overweight:

∾ avoid sweetened drinks
∾ avoid rewarding good behavior with sweets
∾ avoid eating in front of the TV (All meals and snacks should be served at the table.)

- avoid pressuring your child to clean his plate
- avoid giving small children large portions
- and eat fruits and vegetables on a regular basis

If you can do these things for your child, she is unlikely to become overweight.

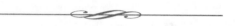

## *Summary*

If you want to avoid conflict at the table and help your child develop healthy habits, follow these guidelines.

1. Eat together at the table and allow your child to serve her own plate.
2. Don't force a child to eat. Respect her ability to self-regulate food intake whether she is fat, thin, or just right.
3. When your child refuses food, don't give in and offer junk foods so she will eat.
4. If a child refuses all foods except a few unhealthy foods, simply do not buy those foods.
5. Adjust portion size to the child. Don't serve kids adult-sized portions.
6. Don't be overly restrictive with food choices, especially at parties, celebrations, and times spent with friends. While junk foods and sweet drinks should not be available on a daily basis, kids don't need to eat perfectly all the time.

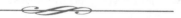

# CHAPTER 5

# Teens

## *Fostering Independence and Healthy Choices*

L ike it or not, as kids become teens and adults, the responsibility for choosing healthy foods shifts out of parents' hands. This is often a time of conflict as teens struggle to make independent decisions while parents have trouble relinquishing control. Conflicts can be especially heated when the parent doesn't feel the teen is making good decisions, or when the teen feels that the parent is being rigid. Most teens want to make their own choices.

On the other hand, many teens try to avoid assuming the daunting responsibility for their own nutritional welfare. These folks end up falling victim to America's vast supply of fast foods and convenience products. Foods like pizza, burgers, and fries are easy to like, easy to obtain, and socially accepted by teen peers. Without guidance, these foods will become staples in a teenager's diet.

A child who has grown up eating fruits and vegetables at the family table will be less vulnerable to the influences of our fast food nation and will likely return to healthy eating practices, but all teens need help and support from their parents to transition into Savvy Eating.

*A child who has grown up eating fruits and vegetables at the family table will be less vulnerable to the influences of our fast food nation and will likely return to healthy eating practices, but all teens need help and support from their parents to transition into Savvy Eating.*

## Teens Need Independence

By the time children become teenagers, they have developed most of their food preferences. However, in their efforts to be independent, teens often develop new eating habits that may be very different from their parents'. For example, a teenager may become a vegetarian for philosophical reasons, they may jump on the fad diet bandwagon because they've become overly concerned with their weight, or they may adopt ultra-strict diets in order to obtain increased athletic performance.

> *In their efforts to be independent, teens often develop new eating habits that may be very different from their parents'. For example, a teenager may become a vegetarian for philosophical reasons, they may jump on the fad diet bandwagon because they've become overly concerned with their weight, or they may adopt ultra-strict diets in order to obtain increased athletic performance.*

When a teen makes a decision about his eating habits, it's comparable to making a decision about his extracurricular activities. Dad may have dreamed that his son would follow in his footsteps and play baseball, but the son's passion may be swim team, tennis, or theater. Think of how hollow the son's victories in swimming would be without Dad's support or how empty his accomplishments in baseball would be if he played only to please his father. So often a child's ambitions, tastes, and desires are different from his parents'. Nevertheless, it's important for a teen to pursue his own legitimate interests. In turn, every teen needs his parents' support and understanding, not necessarily his parents' agreement.

While it's important to respect a teen's independence, it's equally important to continue to provide fruits, vegetables, healthy proteins, and whole grains as a part of a balanced diet. It's also critical to insist on eating at the family table whenever possible. The parents' job is to provide healthy food even if the teen has a history of being a picky eater. It's the teenager's job to eat it. Unless your teen adopts an eating style that is dangerous, try to support his decision. Sometimes it's necessary to turn to a third party, like the teen's doctor, for guidance.

## INDEPENDENT THINKERS OFTEN BOYCOTT MEAT

If your teen refuses meat, support his decision by serving more plant-based proteins like nuts, milk, or rice and beans to ensure that he is getting enough protein. The whole family will benefit from eating less meat. A vegetarian diet is a healthy choice for your family members as long as you know how to get complete proteins at each meal (See chapter 11 to learn more about protein). Because vegetarian diets are often deficient in calcium, iron, zinc, and B vitamins, it's wise to take a vitamin and mineral supplement and have three servings of dairy calcium or a milk substitute daily. Families that are vegetarian due to cultural beliefs are often adept at combining proteins because they prepare traditional time-tested ethnic dishes to get adequate nutrition. First generation vegetarians are at increased risk of nutritional deficiency and could benefit from consulting a dietitian.

### Savvy Eating Tips: Helping Teens Make Wise Choices

You can't tell a teenager what to do anymore than you can tell a toddler. What you **can** do is:

- offer a variety of healthy foods
- let your teen serve his own plate
- insist on eating at the family table whenever schedules allow
- offer him food choices and the opportunity to help plan or prepare meals
- respect his burgeoning sense of independence and support reasonable nutritional preferences
- be alert for signs of eating disorders (excessive weight loss, preoccupation with food or weight, refusal to eat with others, social isolation, dissatisfaction with self image, fatigue, hair loss, loss of menses, and visiting the bathroom frequently and for prolonged lengths of time after meals)

What you **can't** do is:

- make him eat the nutritious food you have prepared

## DON'T SQUELCH AN ADVENTUROUS SPIRIT

Teens often branch out and try new foods that their parents wouldn't think of eating. If your teen decides to eat tofu, seaweed, quinoa, or wheatgrass juice, learn more about them yourself. You might find a new health food! If your teen decides to eat more fruits and vegetables to get more antioxidants, make sure you have an ample supply of healthy produce in the refrigerator even if you don't eat it. If he decides to give up junk food, make healthy foods available by using some of the food preparation techniques found in this book. Sometimes enthusiastic teens can help the whole family to eat better. Enlist your teenager's help in shopping, meal planning, and preparing food. These are skills that your teen will need for independent living.

# CHALLENGES SPECIFIC TO TEENS

## TEEN EATING MACHINES

Teens are notorious for consuming enormous amounts of food. At the peak of growth (around eleven to thirteen for girls and fourteen to sixteen for boys), girls need to eat around 2,200 calories a day, and boys need about 3,000. Teens in sports often need more. That means that some teenage boys can easily eat twice as much as a small adult woman! When hunger strikes, teens will often consume large quantities of whatever is available. If healthy foods are available when teens need to eat, then that is what they will eat.

*When hunger strikes, teens will often consume large quantities of whatever is available. If healthy foods are available when teens need to eat, then that is what they will eat.*

Don't keep chips, pretzels, cookies, crackers, and other junk foods in the house for snacks. These foods are easy to pig out on, leaving little room for nutritious foods that growing teens need. Stock up on fruit, yogurt, nuts, whole-grain cereals, skim milk, peanut butter, and whole-grain bread. Let your teen know which leftovers can be eaten as snacks. A leftover salad, bean burrito, or pasta dish is a much better snack than a bag or two of chips. Rather than empty calories, your teen will get nutrients that he needs. Teen diets are often deficient in calcium, iron, vitamin A, and vitamin C. Snacks should include at least one of these nutrients.

### Savvy Eating Info: Examples of Foods High in Nutrients that Teens Need

| High iron foods | High calcium foods | Foods high in Vitamin A | Foods high in vitamin C |
|---|---|---|---|
| Beans | Skim milk | Orange or yellow fruits like cantaloupe, apricots, mangoes, and nectarines; | Broccoli and other dark green veggies |
| Iron-fortified cereals | Yogurt | | |
| | Fortified soy milk | | Peppers |
| Chicken, beef, pork | Fortified fruit juice | Orange or yellow vegetables like carrots and squash; | Oranges and other citrus fruits |
| Nuts and sunflower seeds | Fortified tofu | | Melons |
| | Cheese | Tomatoes; | Berries |
| Dried plums and apricots | | Watermelon; Red bell peppers; Broccoli | Potatoes (not chips or fries) |

## TEENS NEED TO FIT IN

Just as most teens feel the need to wear clothes that are acceptable to their peers, they may feel the need to eat in a way that is acceptable to their peers. This is not a need born of logic, but nevertheless, it's an integral part of many teens' social lives. While it's not my intent to encourage anyone to go with the flow just to gain social acceptance, it's wise to cut your teen some slack when he wants to eat pizza or fast food with his friends. As long as he is not eating fast food more than two or three times a week and does eat at least one meal at the family table most days, allow him some freedom to choose.

## THE NEED FOR BREAKFAST

Unfortunately, teens' demanding schedules make healthy eating a challenge. Middle and high school students often leave the house for school before eight a.m., with some leaving as early as six! About half of those teens skip breakfast on a regular basis. Some claim there's no time to eat. Others say they just aren't hungry first thing in the morning. Quite a few skip breakfast on the mistaken assumption that it will help them lose weight. Make no mistake! *Breakfast is essential.* School performance, driving ability, general health, sports performance, and mood all suffer when breakfast is skipped.

*Make no mistake! Breakfast is essential. School performance, driving ability, general health, sports performance, and mood all suffer when breakfast is skipped.*

Breakfast also helps prevent obesity as explained in chapter 16. Those who have too little time to sit and eat a bowl of cereal can eat a granola bar or drink a milk- or soy-based breakfast drink. A liquid breakfast is better than no breakfast. A large percentage of teens don't get enough calcium in their diets. Adding a calcium source (like milk, yogurt, or fortified-juice or cereal bars) at breakfast puts them well on their way to getting the three or more servings of calcium-containing foods that they need each day.

Unconventional breakfasts are fine. If your teenager wants leftover pizza or lasagna for breakfast, let him. While there are more nutritious things to eat, at least he's starting the day with enough calories and some protein.

*Unconventional breakfasts are fine. If your teenager wants leftover pizza or lasagna for breakfast, let him. While there are more nutritious things to eat, at least he's starting the day with enough calories and some protein.*

Daily fast food breakfasts, however, are not acceptable. In this case "fast food" is a misnomer. Don't fool yourself. No one can get in the car, go through a busy drive-through, and eat a huge biscuit in less time than they can grab a yogurt from the refrigerator.

Those who aren't hungry or are nauseated by food first thing in the morning probably need to eat breakfast even more than most folks. Those who have experienced morning sickness with pregnancy understand how these breakfast skippers feel. When energy needs go up as in times of teenage growth or pregnancy, overnight fasting causes the blood sugar to drop. Because you're sleeping rather than eating, your body shifts to a lower metabolic state or starvation mode. The feeling of hunger is decreased, but the need for calories is not. Low blood sugar can make some people experience nausea.

Having a protein-containing snack like peanuts or a glass of milk at bedtime can help level out blood sugar through the night and can alleviate morning nausea. Avoiding sweets with the last meal of the day can help too. If nausea persists, start slow in the morning with a glass of milk or juice, but don't give up on breakfast. It would be better to eat a granola bar on the bus or eat a piece of fruit between classes than skip breakfast entirely.

# Diet Dilemmas

Many teenage girls begin to diet as natural feminine curves start to develop at puberty. Because pop culture highly prizes the thin androgynous physique, many girls mistake their new curves for excess fat. While only 15 percent of teenage girls are overweight, 70 percent of teenage girls express a desire to lose weight.

On the flip side, athletes often want to force their bodies to look like those on the covers of muscle and fitness magazines. These aren't realistic goals for most people, and no amount of protein supplementation and fat deprivation will make most teenage bodies look like Arnold Schwarzenegger.

While athletes' bodies do need extra calories, protein, iron, calcium, vitamins, and other nutrients, teen athletes don't need the protein supplements sold in health food stores. Unless they're on a low-protein, vegetarian diet, the Savvy Eating Plan described in this book plus a daily multivitamin with iron and calcium will provide excellent nutrition for the average teen athlete. By consuming more calories to supply his energy needs, an athlete who eats a source of complete protein at each meal and as part of most snacks will automatically get plenty of protein for his growing body.

If your teenager decides to go on a specific diet, don't minimize the importance of his decision. Your child is feeling angst over some aspect

## Savvy Eating Info: Supplements and Vitamins

### Are nutritional supplements safe for teens?

That depends on the supplement. A multivitamin containing no more than the recommended daily allowance (RDA) of vitamins and minerals is a safe and time-tested beneficial practice. If your teen does not eat meat on a daily basis, then the supplement should contain iron. If your teen does not drink at least three servings of milk or eat at least three servings of calcium fortified foods, the supplement should contain calcium too.

### Mega doses of vitamins and minerals are risky at best.

Overdoses of some vitamins and minerals like vitamin A and iron are toxic. Mega doses of other supplements have little benefit. The body can only absorb a limited amount of most vitamins and minerals. Mega doses of vitamin C, for example, are not used by the body and just make expensive urine.

### Don't be fooled by the "all natural" claim.

Just because the manufacturer claims that a product is natural, it does not in any way imply that the product is safe. Cyanide and arsenic are "all natural" as well as deadly. Most major brands of vitamins in the U.S. are safe, but it's a good idea to consult ConsumerLab.com for safety testing information.

### Are herbal supplements and remedies safe?

Some are; some aren't. Be sure to let your doctor know if you're taking any herbs or supplements. Not all traditionally trained physicians are knowledgeable about the supplement you want to take, so make sure you talk with a doctor who's informed before starting an alternative remedy.

Steroid muscle building hormones (like androstenedione) and amphetamines (uppers or pep pills) are dangerous and should not be used. Many nutritional supplements marketed to athletes as performance enhancers have been shown to be contaminated with steroids and toxic chemicals. Others just don't deliver the desired results. Remember, the government does not regulate dietary supplements safety or health claims. Buyer beware!

of his health and body. He may need to lose some weight or merely want a more ideal physique. If you demonstrate to your child that you can't see things from his point of view by discounting his concerns, he'll be less likely to listen to your advice or come to you for help.

If your child wants to diet, acknowledge his feelings even if you don't agree. He may hide his dieting from you if you show him that you don't understand the way he feels. Make sure his goals are realistic. No teen should try to live on 500 calories a day, eat only grapefruit, or shun carbohydrates entirely to lose weight. Extreme diets do not result in healthy weight loss and have great potential for harm.

Even less extreme diets can be harmful. Magazines popular with teens often promote diets that shun foods perceived to be "fattening foods." Unfortunately, these foods are often the foods that teens need most like calcium-rich milk, protein-rich meat, and healthy fat and protein-containing nuts.

Show your teen support by educating him as well as yourself about his nutritional needs. Any teen who decides to make a dramatic change in his diet during this critical period of growth should have a check-up with a physician. You need to make sure that your teen's diet is safe, then back off and let your teen eat.

# When Not to Back Off

Allowing your teen the right to make his own choices does not mean that you don't need to watch for signs of danger. Eating disorders are common, especially in girls. Anorexia nervosa (severe weight loss resulting

---

### *Savvy Eating Info: Signs of Eating Disorders*

Anorexia
- Marked weight loss
- Loss of menstrual periods
- Compulsive or excessive exercising
- Odd or obsessive eating behaviors
- Depressed mood
- Perceiving oneself as fat in spite of weight loss
- Denial that behavior is abnormal

Bulimia
- Frequent weight loss or gain
- Episodes of eating huge quantities of food
- Fear of losing control of eating, being unable to stop
- Frequent severe dieting or fasting
- Low self-esteem, shame
- Awareness that behavior is abnormal
- Depression

from unrealistic body image and extreme caloric restriction) and bulimia (characterized by binging on large amounts of food, then purging by vomiting, using laxatives or extreme dieting) commonly develop in the mid-teen years. If your child shows signs of an eating disorder, professional intervention is mandatory.

Both anorexics and bulimics may purge (laxative abuse or vomiting after meals), but can be very secretive. Loss of tooth enamel can result from frequent forced vomiting. Your child's doctor or dentist may pick this up.

## *Summary*

The teen years can be challenging. It's a time to make sure you maintain communication with your child and refrain from making judgments. Your teen has the best chance of developing and continuing healthy eating practices if you follow these guidelines:

1. Be aware that teens need to make independent decisions that reflect their social, ethical, and taste preferences. It's time for you to gradually render control.
2. Teens' preferences are often very different from their parents. Support their decisions, however different from yours, as long as they are safe.
3. You can't force a teen to eat well, but it is your job to provide him with nutritious food and a family table on a daily basis.
4. Provide breakfast daily.
5. Teens have special nutritional needs, including an increased need for calcium, iron, calories, and vitamins A and C. Provide snacks and meals with these issues in mind.
6. Teens face many social and emotional pressures that affect their nutrition. Be understanding of their desire to diet, but make sure that their goals are realistic and that dieting teens are seen by a health professional at least annually.
7. Be alert for signs of eating disorders.

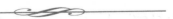

# CHAPTER 6

# Savvy Eating Grows Up but Not Old

In America, growing up is synonymous with having the freedom to choose how we live our lives, including how we eat, but that doesn't make it any easier to eat well. Americans have too many choices. Whole aisles of grocery stores are filled with low nutrient density snack foods that are convenient and cheap, and yet most adults can ill afford to eat these foods.

> *By the time we reach our twenties, growth has stopped and our caloric needs decline, but our requirements for most nutrients remain the same.*

By the time we reach our twenties, growth has stopped and our caloric needs decline, but our requirements for most nutrients remain the same. We need just as many vitamins and micronutrients from less food. That means less room for low nutrient density foods if we want to maintain a healthy weight. Therefore, we need to make better choices if we want to be healthy.

## Too Busy to Eat Well

Adults are pulled in many different directions. Work, travel, stress, and family obligations take priority and eating becomes something that happens along the way. Even healthy eaters face challenges as they marry and, for better or for worse, combine two different sets of eating habits.

Consider the following scenario:

Mary was a healthy eater and an athlete in college. After marrying David, her habits changed. While David played team sports in college, he never got in the habit of exercising just for the sake of health and wasn't very patient when Mary did. When Mary would fit in a jog after work, David, an avid grill master and meat-and-potatoes man, would be relaxing with a beer while flipping juicy eight-ounce steaks. Tired and grateful to have tasty food set in front of her, Mary would enjoy David's steaks and beer and resolve to eat the crisper-full of wilting veggies another night.

Healthy stir-fried tofu and veggies, her college staple, gradually became a thing of the past. How could she complain? David even did a lot of the shopping and kept the pantry full, albeit full of chips, soda, and cookies. Even if only one partner has poor eating habits, just having junk food around the house will pose a challenge to most healthy eaters.

As adults move into the family stage of life, picky children can put a damper on the variety and nutrition in a family's diet. Mary and David soon became the proud parents of a little girl and boy. Mary and David continued to work full time. Life was hectic, but happy. Fast food and frozen diners became the house special. Life was too busy to stop and enjoy food, besides the kids wouldn't touch her tofu and veggies after David complained, saying, "not health food again!"

Preparing blander foods with kid appeal can lead to a monotonous and unsatisfying diet. Adults who eat chicken nuggets and fries instead of dishes like marinated grilled chicken with asparagus, broccoli, and carrots are likely to gain weight and lose valuable nutrients too. Weight gain is especially pronounced for those parents who indulge in the "parents' fifth food group," your child's leavings.

> *Weight gain is especially pronounced for those parents who indulge in the "parents' fifth food group," your child's leavings.*

Long work hours challenge even the healthiest of intentions. David always enjoyed a good healthy breakfast. But now that his boss was urging him to work later hours and show up earlier in order to get a promotion, he found himself burning the candle at both ends. When faced with the choice between twenty more minutes of sleep or cereal, he skipped breakfast.

David, like all breakfast skippers, was vulnerable to doughnuts in the break room, a latte on the go, and snacks from the ever-present vending machine. Fast-food menus and vending machines are not known for their nutritious selections. Even those who can pass up the available temptation often arrive at lunchtime famished, and David was no exception.

> *Now that you're on your way to becoming a Savvy Eater, you will learn how to resist the temptation of junk food by planning ahead and filling up on better-tasting, nutritious food.*

Fast-food lunches are too easy to obtain since most of America is dotted with fast-food chains on every corner. Even if you can't leave work long enough to spin through the drive-through, chances are that someone in the office will pick up a burger and fries for you on their way.

Now that you're on your way to becoming a Savvy Eater, you will learn how to resist the temptation of junk food by planning ahead and filling up on better-tasting, nutritious food. See chapters 18 through 29 for meal plans, shopping guides, and simple recipes.

# Dining with Stress

## EATING OUT

The fast food lunch is not the only challenge working adults face. Business lunches and dinners can sometimes mean even worse nutrition. For example, after his promotion, David often entertained clients at upscale steak houses. The meals were heavy on refined carbohydrates, saturated fats, and calories. While many of the meals did include a salad, it was usually topped with a generous amount of creamy dressing. (A quarter cup often contains over 300 calories!) These meals usually included both alcohol (a 130-calorie cocktail) and dessert (a 700-calorie slice of cherry cheese cake). Too much! The salad, dessert, and cocktail alone contained more than a third of David's daily calorie needs. Need I even mention the large New York strip and baked potato with butter and sour cream?

Business meals and workday lunches are often eaten under stress, too. Whoever thought that trying to close a business deal while choking down rich food was a good idea? Eating with stress and distraction makes you less satisfied with your meal. Sometimes David would find himself raiding the break room mid-afternoon even after a 1,500-calorie fancy meal. That was stress, not hunger talking.

*Savvy Eaters will learn to choose restaurant foods that are good for them, while avoiding overeating (see chapter 15).*

Savvy Eaters will learn to choose restaurant foods that are good for them, while avoiding overeating (see chapter 15).

## EATING ON THE RUN AND EATING ALONE

The diets of those who travel for business also suffer the consequences of fast-food and business lunches three times a day. They suffer from eating alone too. David would mindlessly wolf down meals on the go while he was traveling on business. He would usually do it in a rush while working or even driving back from a fast-food joint. That's a prescription for indigestion, and soon David was taking antacids.

Whether you're out of town, in the office, or at home alone, eating by yourself can present its own challenges. If you pause to enjoy your food and eat mindfully, eating alone can be a satisfying and relaxing experience. Savvy Eaters will learn to recognize their stress triggers and avoid mindless eating (see chapter 7).

THE LURE OF COMFORT FOODS

Many adults find themselves eating comfort foods in excess when they're under stress. Mary was a single parent for most of the week since David was out of town on business so much of the time. She would juggle her work schedule to get the kids to games and practices. She would come home feeling exhausted and frazzled.

*If you pause to enjoy your food and eat mindfully, eating alone can be a satisfying and relaxing experience. Savvy Eaters will learn to recognize their stress triggers and avoid mindless eating (see chapter 7).*

When her life felt out of control, she searched for sources of pleasure she could control. Treating herself to comfort food like chocolates and ice cream seemed like a reasonable indulgence for a busy person who has given her all at the office and on the home front, until it spiraled out of control. Mary had gained almost thirty pounds in the last five years. Loss of control over her eating habits made the stress situation for Mary even worse.

It's easy to see how healthy young adults can end up like Mary and David even without the ringer your metabolism throws in as we age.

## Your Metabolism Ain't What It Used to Be

Adults face not only lifestyle challenges as we age, but also physical challenges, to the point that it sometimes feels like our bodies are turning against us! Most of the physical changes that occur in adulthood are subtle and have a way of sneaking up on us. Our basal metabolic rate decreases about 2 to 5 percent every ten years starting at age thirty.

*Our basal metabolic rate decreases about 2 to 5 percent every ten years starting at age thirty.*

That doesn't sound like much, but over time, it can have a big impact on your health. As we grow older, the metabolic rate decreases even further, about 10 percent a decade after age fifty.

A woman who needs 2,100 calories at age twenty will only need 2,000 calories at age thirty-five and only 1,800 calories by age fifty. For men, the decrease is more dramatic. A twenty-year-old who needs 2,900 calories will need 500 fewer calories a day by age fifty.

If you consider that eating one hundred extra calories a day can mean a weight gain of ten pounds over a year, then you see how easy it would be to put on an extra twenty, fifty, or even one hundred pounds over a lifetime. A thirty-five year old who eats just as she did at twenty-five might be fifty pounds overweight. The decrease in metabolic rate is due in large part to the gradual loss of muscle tissue as we age.

The average person over thirty-five loses a half pound of muscle a year. Muscle burns more calories than fat. The more muscle you lose, the slower your metabolism, and the easier it is for you to gain weight. Adults who don't continue to do muscle-building exercise will need to eat less and less to stay the same size.

The Savvy Eating Plan will help you eat less without feeling deprived by slowly downsizing your portions while increasing satisfaction.

> *The more muscle you lose, the slower your metabolism, and the easier it is for you to gain weight. Adults who don't continue to do muscle-building exercise will need to eat less and less to stay the same size.*

## Some Healthy Foods Don't Agree with Us Anymore

### LACTOSE INTOLERANCE

Our bodies can let us down in other ways too. By middle age, some degree of lactose intolerance is the norm. You might gradually start noticing that you have more gas and bloating than you used to. You might even develop intermittent diarrhea.

The culprit may be lactose, the carbohydrate found in milk. We often lose the ability to digest lactose as we get older. Friendly bacteria that live in our guts can help the lactose intolerant digest milk, but antibiotics and diarrhea can decrease the population of these helpful organisms, leaving us unable to drink a glass of milk without gastrointestinal distress.

The Savvy Eating Plan is flexible, allowing those who cannot digest dairy to get plenty of protein and calcium by substituting soy, rice, and nut products for dairy (see chapter 11).

### HEARTBURN

Americans spend millions of dollars a year trying to alleviate this common problem with antacids and other drugs used to treat gastroesophageal reflux and peptic ulcer disease. While fried foods, stress, and over eating are common triggers that everyone should avoid, some healthy foods like tomatoes, citrus fruits, and hot peppers are also triggers. Following the Savvy Eating Plan can help reduce the need for antacids and other medications and for many reflux sufferers, allow them to enjoy some of their favorite healthy foods (sometimes even chocolate and coffee) again.

### CONSTIPATION

This common problem plagues more adults than care to admit it. If your bowel movements are ever hard or lumpy, you are constipated, no matter how regular you are! Constipation commonly causes cramping and painful gas. Many people give up on eating a high-fiber healthy diet because they're so uncomfortable with gas and bloating. The problem is not so much the bulky food, but the constipation that was there first. When you're accustomed to a diet of refined foods, your stool is compact and slow moving. When you eat a high-fiber diet, your stool is large, soft, and moves quickly through the intestine. When a high-fiber meal follows a habit of refined foods, it can spell trouble. Gas builds up, but can't escape. This causes pain and bloating. Savvy Eaters learn to gradually and consistently add whole grains, fruits, and vegetables to their diet to avoid constipation, gas, and discomfort (see chapter 10).

*Savvy Eaters learn to gradually and consistently add whole grains, fruits, and vegetables to their diet to avoid constipation, gas, and discomfort (see chapter 10).*

## Special Challenges that Come with Age

The elderly face even more nutritional challenges. While young adults are often too busy to eat well, the elderly sometimes have too much time on their hands. That makes it easy to place too much importance on food. Some elderly people face decreased income, decreased mobility, impaired hearing and vision, as well as medical disabilities, which can leave eating as one of their few remaining daily pleasures. It isn't easy to eat smaller quantities of food if eating is the day's main source of pleasure.

The Savvy Eater will discover that eating at the family table benefits all generations by placing the emphasis on the social aspects of eating rather than on the consumption of large quantities of decadent food.

### HOW TO HELP THE ELDERLY OVERCOME CHALLENGES TO HEALTHY EATING

Whether you're getting older or you find yourself caring for aged parents, the following tips can help.

- ∾ Tooth loss makes it hard to chew healthy salads, raw vegetables, and nuts. Decreased salivary and digestive enzymes make it difficult to digest some of the same foods. Switching from salads to pureed vegetable soups can help keep plenty of antioxidants in the diet. Adding peanut and nut butters to baked goods is a good way to make healthy nuts more edible.

∾ Decreased appetite is common, as is disorientation. Eating at the family table can help with both issues. The family table may mean eating with a group of friends, neighbors, or a church group rather than actual relatives. Elderly people who are showing signs of disorientation need to eat with others. Take advantage of community support systems, Meals on Wheels, and hired help if needed.

∾ The elderly often suffer from dehydration due to decreased sensitivity to thirst. Offer soups, fresh fruit, and water frequently to help alleviate this situation.

∾ Decreased sense of smell and taste can lead to over-salting of food, and in some cases, lack of interest in eating. The family table helps here too. Eating with others stimulates appetite. Family members, friends, or caretakers can make sure the salt shaker stays off the table.

∾ Decreased coordination or vision can lead to overuse of convenience foods and fast food because preparing foods can become difficult if not dangerous. Using Savvy Eating techniques to prepare foods in advance (and perhaps in the company of relatives or friends) can help the elderly stock their pantries with easy-prep nutritious foods.

∾ Illness and medications often add restrictions to diets. Savvy Eating involves low-salt, low glycemic load, high-fiber foods without artificial additives that complement the prescribed diets of many older adults.

---

### Savvy Eating Tips: Healthy Aging

By 2015, almost one-third of our population will be over sixty-five. Unfortunately, there's no miracle elixir to cure aging. While aging can't be prevented entirely, the Savvy Eating Plan will certainly slow down the clock and help us age well. Eating smaller meals, keeping weight down, controlling glycemic load, getting plenty of antioxidants while avoiding toxic foods is the only way to slow the degeneration and disease associated with aging. Many of the medical ills like heart disease, stroke, cancer and diabetes that are associated with aging can be prevented or improved through Savvy Eating, even if you're not an avid exerciser.

## *Summary*

Eating well can be a challenge at any age. So many Americans find there are too many choices, too much stress, or too little time to make healthy eating their habit and just give up. As our bodies age, we are threatened by food intolerances, reflux, constipation, and other ailments that further challenge our eating habits. Take heart! If you're ready to feel confident about your food choices, to make healthy eating easier, and to improve your health, read on.

In the next chapters, you will take an honest look at your current eating habits and look for simple ways to improve them. Then you'll take an in-depth look at how to achieve optimal nutrition. You'll find information on how to shop for, prepare, and enjoy the foods that you need to be eating. Savvy Eating will be easy when you know how to incorporate the principles of good nutrition into your life. Here are some examples of what you're about to learn:

1. To use portion control to avoid weight gain as you age (chapter 12).
2. To anticipate your needs and avoid fast-food and junk food by being prepared. To learn how to have healthy snacks, wholesome lunches, and nutritious fast dinners at your fingertips (chapters 10, 13, and 18).
3. To choose selections wisely when eating out (chapter 15).
4. To enjoy your food and gain satisfaction by eating mindfully (chapter 6).
5. To incorporate highly nutritious food into your diet painlessly in part two of the book. Great menu plans and recipes will make Savvy Eating a part of your life.

# CHAPTER 7

# Evaluate Yourself

## *Nothing but the Truth*

The first step in your journey toward a healthy diet is to honestly evaluate your current habits. The best way to do this is by keeping a food journal. It's the easiest way to step back and look at which foods you need to eat more often and which ones you need to eat less often. Teens and kids over eight can keep their own journals.

Once you've taken the time to keep a food journal, you're well on your way toward healthy eating. It's a well-known dietary principle that just the act of writing down your eating habits will help improve them.

## Track What You Really Put into Your Stomach

Choose a two-week period to record in a notebook *everything* you *eat* or *drink*. Record the *time* of day the food was eaten, measure and record the *quantity* of food, and *how you felt* before and after eating it. You might feel *starved, hungry, satisfied, full, or stuffed*. Be specific about the amount and type of foods you eat. Be sure to include everything you drink too. Here's a sample daily food journal:

### Savvy Eating Example: Daily Food Journal

| Time | Food | How I felt before | How I felt after |
|------|------|-------------------|------------------|
| 7:30 a.m. | 1 slice white toast with 2 teaspoons margarine 12 ounces coffee with 3 tablespoons whole milk 8 ounces orange juice | Hungry | Satisfied |
| 10:00 a.m. | ½ (5 ounce) package M&M candy 8 ounces coffee with 3 tablespoons whole milk | Hungry | Satisfied |

| 1:45 p.m. | 1 fried chicken filet sandwich with white bun large ( 6 ounce) fries with 2 tablespoons ketchup 24 ounces diet Coke | Starved | Full |
|---|---|---|---|
| 7:15 p.m. | 2 cups spaghetti with ¾ cup meat sauce ½ cup parmesan cheese Salad with 1 cup iceberg lettuce, ¼ cup tomato, ¼ cup carrots, ¼ cup cucumber, and 3 tablespoons bottled Italian dressing 5 ounces red wine 8 ounces water 1 slice of cheesecake (¹⁄₁₀ of cake) | Starved | Stuffed |
| 9:45 p.m. | 5 ounces pretzels 12 ounces Coke | Satisfied | Satisfied |

Once you've kept a food journal, see how well you've accomplished the main goals of healthy eating. Think of ways you can substitute, add, or eliminate foods to make your diet healthier. Keep your journal with you as you read the rest of this book to learn simple ways to make improvements in your diet. Once you've mastered the main goals of healthy eating, then you can work on some of the finer points.

When evaluating your journal, there are several questions to ask yourself:

### What Healthy Foods Do I Need to Eat More of?

Most of us need to eat more fruits and vegetables (five to thirteen servings a day), healthy fats, and whole grains. Many need to include more calcium sources (two to three servings a day), whether it's from dairy products or supplements. Use the summary points at the end of each chapter as a guide to what you should be eating.

It's also important to include a *variety* of foods in your diet in order to get enough micronutrients. A steady diet of the same nutritious foods every day may not be sufficient to keep you healthy.

### What Types of Foods Do I Need to limit?

The most common ones are full-fat dairy products, red meat, processed foods, high GI foods, and foods containing trans fats. Learn how to avoid these in the next few chapters.

## DO I NEED TO DECREASE THE NUMBER OF CALORIES I EAT?

The answer is yes if you're overweight. The best person to determine whether you're overweight is your doctor, but adults can determine your body mass index (BMI) by looking it up in the chart on page 62.

The BMI is not a perfect measure of healthy body weight. It tends to overestimate the appropriate weight for the elderly who have diminished muscle mass and underestimate the appropriate weight for those who are extremely muscular. In spite of its shortcomings, BMI is a good place to start. A BMI of nineteen to twenty-four is considered healthy for adults. A BMI eighteen or under would be underweight. A BMI twenty-five to thirty is overweight, and a BMI over thirty is considered obese.

The standards for children's BMIs are based on age and require special charts to interpret. Your child's pediatrician will calculate your child's BMI at each well visit. If you don't know your child's BMI, ask your pediatrician to calculate it and explain the result.

If you're underweight or of normal weight and are trying to maintain healthy weight, do not count calories. For those trying to lose weight, it's helpful to be aware of the relative calorie counts of favorite foods, so portion size and frequency of indulgence in these foods can be adjusted. Knowing that a single slice of cheesecake has over 700 calories might convince you to eat half a piece or choose a 150-calorie scoop of ice cream instead. While the number of calories you consume in relation to the number you burn ultimately determines whether or not you maintain a healthy weight, counting calories is a cumbersome task that can take the enjoyment out of eating. For most of us, it's not very helpful either, since we don't know exactly how many calories we burn in a day. What we do know is that if you're overweight, you need to eat fewer calories than you do now without undue sacrifice or starvation.

> *Knowing that a single slice of cheesecake has over 700 calories might convince you to eat half a piece or choose a 150-calorie scoop of ice cream instead.*

## AM I EATING TO SATISFY HUNGER OR FOR OTHER REASONS?

If you were "hungry" when you started eating, and "satisfied," not "full," or "stuffed" when you finished, you're following appropriate hunger cues when you eat. If you were "full" or "stuffed" after eating, you are overeating.

> *If you were "full" or "stuffed" after eating, you are overeating.*

# Satiety Awareness

Cultivating awareness of satiety is one of the key components of Savvy Eating. Pausing to assess whether you're starved, hungry, satisfied, full, or stuffed after each meal or snack is as important, or possibly more important, than writing down the foods you eat when you keep your food journal.

*Cultivating awareness of satiety is one of the key components of Savvy Eating.*

Slowing down to enjoy food in a pleasant location can help you avoid overeating. Eating in the car, during a meeting, or even with a demanding young family can be stressful. Eating a meal under duress can make you feel unsatisfied even if you have eaten enough calories. You may find yourself seeking something else to eat after such a meal even though you're full. Strive to eat in as peaceful a situation as possible and sit down and enjoy your food. Enjoying food is a basic human right.

If you were "starved" when you started eating, you're either waiting too long between meals or eating too many high GI foods. (High GI foods cause you to feel hungry because their calories end up stored as fat rather than used for energy.) When you wait until you're starving to eat, you're more likely to pick up and eat the most convenient food you can find. A bag of chips is opened and gone before you can head out the door to buy a salad; so making healthy foods available is key. Starving yourself (waiting too long between eating) also causes you to overeat once you finally eat again because you tend to eat quickly, packing down lots of calories before your stomach has time to communicate to your brain that you're full. (This usually takes about twenty minutes). Starving yourself also causes the body's metabolism to slow down so you burn the calories you do eat less efficiently. This is why those who skip breakfast often become overweight.

*Starving yourself also causes the body's metabolism to slow down so you burn the calories you do eat less efficiently.*

Eating more fruits, vegetables, and whole grains can help you stay satisfied longer, largely because they take a long time to digest. Having some protein at each meal or snack helps you feel satisfied longer too.

# Cravings

Eating a variety of healthy unprocessed foods may actually help decrease food cravings. Many people—especially pregnant women, women with premenstrual syndrome, and those with proven deficiencies such as iron deficiency—have strong cravings. People with iron deficiency, for example, often have "pica," which is the craving to eat non-nutritive substances like ice or dirt. Premenstrual women often crave chocolate; pregnant women often crave oranges or red meat. Some of these cravings make sense: Pregnant women need lots of iron (found in red meat) and folate (found in oranges), and premenstrual women may need extra magnesium (found in chocolate). Other cravings like eating dirt or ice make absolutely no nutritional sense whatsoever. What does make sense is that we have cravings when our body is deficient in some nutrient. The missing nutrient may be something very basic like water or overall calories. Sometimes we have cravings when we're just hungry or thirsty. Or we may crave something less obvious like selenium, an important nutrient in immune functions and cancer prevention found in nuts, etc. It may be that we have an imbalance between the amount of toxic substances we ingest and the amount of antioxidants we need to neutralize them.

We are far from being able to translate our body's cravings into a grocery list of what our body needs. There are currently no studies to confirm that cravings equal deficiency or imbalance, but it does make sense to include a variety of nutrient and antioxidant-rich foods in our diet. When you have a craving, think about how you have been eating lately. What nutrient might be missing from your diet? If you crave something that is good for you like strawberries, then indulge. If your craving is for a hot fudge sundae, chances are your body doesn't need exactly that. Maybe you haven't been eating whole grains, vegetables, or a dairy source lately. Make an effort to eat what your diet has lacked most recently and see if the craving persists. If it persists, eat a reasonable sized serving of what you crave and don't worry about it.

We have many other reasons for eating when we're not hungry. Sometimes we eat because it's time to eat, even if we're satisfied. Unless food is not going to be available later, wait until you're hungry to eat. Conversely, you shouldn't wait until a set mealtime to eat if you're hungry now.

## Temptation and Overeating

Sometimes we eat because a desirable food becomes available or is seen or smelled. When you see a lucious chocolate cake on the cover of a magazine or worse, on your kitchen counter, you find yourself wanting a slice even if you're not hungry. It is best to keep tempting foods out of sight and even better, out of the house. Simply not purchasing unhealthy foods is the single best way to prevent eating them. This is especially helpful for children who may not be able to resist temptation and wage food battles with their parents to get unhealthy foods.

*"Buffet Syndrome"* is another cause of overeating. Few people are tempted to overeat when faced with a large bowl of plain oatmeal. But when faced with a sumptuous buffet of fruit, pastries, pancakes, omelets, bacon, and doughnuts (and what's more, you've paid for "all you can eat!"), it's difficult not to try a little of every thing. Unfortunately, a little of everything ends up being a lot of calories. When you see a large variety of appealing foods, you're stimulated to want to sample each kind even if you become satisfied before the sampling is done.

You can use "Buffet Syndrome" to your advantage, however. When serving a meal, planning a party, or simply packing your lunch, prepare a variety of foods that you need to eat more of. For example, rather than preparing a large amount of mashed potatoes and green beans for supper, prepare a mixture of roasted root vegetables (potatoes, sweet potatoes, carrots, and onions), and green beans with garlic, and sliced oranges. You're much more likely to eat your necessary five to nine servings of fruits and vegetables if you have a variety on your plate.

By the same token, if you're trying to eat less of a certain type of food, like sweets, only prepare a small quantity of the unhealthy food and avoid going to places that serve a variety of that type of food. For example, if you're going to a buffet restaurant, go to one that offers a wide variety of salads, soups, and vegetables, but serves only ice cream rather than a dessert bar.

## Stress, Boredom, and Overeating

We sometimes eat because we're bored or upset. Eating when bored has an obvious solution that takes willpower to carry out. If you're bored and munchy, find something constructive to do, like exercise. Eating when you're upset is a more complex issue that may require professional help, but sometimes being aware of the reason you're overeating can help put a stop to it.

It's important to slow down. Don't quickly chew and swallow your food (or even worse, swallow your food without adequately chewing). Chewing you food well helps you digest your food more easily and can prevent a common cause of indigestion.

Don't contemplate your next bite until you're finished with the one in your mouth. This will increase satisfaction, improve digestion, and help prevent overeating.

### Savvy Eating Exercise: Eating Mindfully

Have you have ever looked down to find an empty bag of chips in your hand and not honestly remember how all that food made it from the bag to your stomach? Do you find yourself unable to stop picking at the chocolate chip cookie dough ice cream: Just one more spoonful, ooh a chunk! Just a little more chocolate swirl . . . until half the box is gone? Do you ever gulp down your food in anticipation of the next bite rather than enjoying what's in your mouth now? Do you have trouble remembering what you ate for lunch? If you answered "yes" to any of these questions, you need to practice mindful eating. Try this exercise:

1. Place a single raisin or chocolate chip into your mouth. Chew as slowly as possible. Close your eyes, enjoy the flavor and sweetness. Concentrate on the taste rather than thinking about other things.
2. Place a small handful of raisins or chocolate chips in front of you. Repeat the exercise, enjoying as many as you care to eat. Try to enjoy the morsel in your mouth rather than anticipating the next one.
3. Repeat the exercise in front of the TV. Which raisin or chip did you enjoy the most? Which one took you the longest to eat? Chances are the ones eaten in front of the TV were the quickest to go and the least enjoyed. Remind yourself of this exercise whenever you eat.

## Summary

Consider the reasons behind your food choices as you keep your food journal and take notes. Your diet need not be perfect. Nobody knows exactly what a perfect diet would be, but once you understand the basic goals of healthy eating as explained in the next few chapters, you can learn how to avoid many dietary pitfalls. Then it's time to break some old habits and make some new ones.

What matters the most in your overall health is what you do on a day-to-day basis. Eliminating trans fats from your pantry shelves, substituting whole grains for processed foods, eating fish or nuts often in place of red meat, and learning easy and delicious ways to enjoy vegetables every day will make a huge impact on your health. Going out once a week for a burger and fries or enjoying a pastry on Saturday morning will probably have little effect on your overall health if you eat healthy

*The occasional indulgence is the spice of life, but your daily habits are the backbone.*

foods the majority of the time. The occasional indulgence is the spice of life, but your daily habits are the backbone.

When you keep your journal, ask yourself the following questions:

1. What healthy foods do I need to eat more of?
2. What foods do I need to limit?
3. Do I need to eat fewer calories?
4. Am I eating to satisfy hunger or for other reasons?

| Body Mass Index Table | | | | | | | | | | | | | | | | |
|---|---|---|---|---|---|---|---|---|---|---|---|---|---|---|---|---|
| | Normal | | | | | | Overweight | | | | | Obese | | | | |
| BMI | 19 | 20 | 21 | 22 | 23 | 24 | 25 | 26 | 27 | 28 | 29 | 30 | 31 | 32 | 33 | 34 | 35 |
| Height (inches) | | | | | | | Body Weight (pounds) | | | | | | | | | | |
| 58 | 91 | 96 | 100 | 105 | 110 | 115 | 119 | 124 | 129 | 134 | 138 | 143 | 148 | 153 | 158 | 162 | 167 |
| 59 | 94 | 99 | 104 | 109 | 114 | 119 | 124 | 128 | 133 | 138 | 143 | 148 | 153 | 158 | 163 | 168 | 173 |
| 60 | 97 | 102 | 107 | 112 | 118 | 123 | 128 | 133 | 138 | 143 | 148 | 153 | 158 | 163 | 168 | 174 | 179 |
| 61 | 100 | 106 | 111 | 116 | 122 | 127 | 132 | 137 | 143 | 148 | 153 | 158 | 164 | 169 | 174 | 180 | 185 |
| 62 | 104 | 109 | 115 | 120 | 126 | 131 | 136 | 142 | 147 | 153 | 158 | 164 | 169 | 175 | 180 | 186 | 191 |
| 63 | 107 | 113 | 118 | 124 | 130 | 135 | 141 | 146 | 152 | 158 | 163 | 169 | 175 | 180 | 186 | 191 | 197 |
| 64 | 110 | 116 | 122 | 128 | 134 | 140 | 145 | 151 | 157 | 163 | 169 | 174 | 180 | 186 | 192 | 197 | 204 |
| 65 | 114 | 120 | 126 | 132 | 138 | 144 | 150 | 156 | 162 | 168 | 174 | 180 | 186 | 192 | 198 | 204 | 210 |
| 66 | 118 | 124 | 130 | 136 | 142 | 148 | 155 | 161 | 167 | 173 | 179 | 186 | 192 | 198 | 204 | 210 | 216 |
| 67 | 121 | 127 | 134 | 140 | 146 | 153 | 159 | 166 | 172 | 178 | 185 | 191 | 198 | 204 | 211 | 217 | 223 |
| 68 | 125 | 131 | 138 | 144 | 151 | 158 | 164 | 171 | 177 | 184 | 190 | 197 | 203 | 210 | 216 | 223 | 230 |
| 69 | 128 | 135 | 142 | 149 | 155 | 162 | 169 | 176 | 182 | 189 | 196 | 203 | 209 | 216 | 223 | 230 | 236 |
| 70 | 132 | 139 | 146 | 153 | 160 | 167 | 174 | 181 | 188 | 195 | 202 | 209 | 216 | 222 | 229 | 236 | 243 |
| 71 | 136 | 143 | 150 | 157 | 165 | 172 | 179 | 186 | 193 | 200 | 208 | 215 | 222 | 229 | 236 | 243 | 250 |
| 72 | 140 | 147 | 154 | 162 | 169 | 177 | 184 | 191 | 199 | 206 | 213 | 221 | 228 | 235 | 242 | 250 | 258 |
| 73 | 144 | 151 | 159 | 166 | 174 | 182 | 189 | 197 | 204 | 212 | 219 | 227 | 235 | 242 | 250 | 257 | 265 |
| 74 | 148 | 155 | 163 | 171 | 179 | 186 | 194 | 202 | 210 | 218 | 225 | 233 | 241 | 249 | 256 | 264 | 272 |
| 75 | 152 | 160 | 168 | 176 | 184 | 192 | 200 | 208 | 216 | 224 | 232 | 240 | 248 | 256 | 264 | 272 | 279 |
| 76 | 156 | 164 | 172 | 180 | 189 | 197 | 205 | 213 | 221 | 230 | 238 | 246 | 254 | 263 | 271 | 279 | 287 |

Source: Adapted from *Clinical Guidelines on the Identification, Evaluation, and Treatment of Overweight and Obesity in Adults: The Evidence Report.*

# CHAPTER 8

# The Facts on Fat

Now for some good news. We can relax a little bit about the amount of fat in our diets. With the rising tide of obesity in our society, many erroneously assumed that fat in the diet was the main culprit behind the fat on our behinds, so to speak. It's not that simple.

While the *type* of fat we consume plays a vital role in our health, the overall *percentage* of fat in our diets has some wiggle room. When the government made the recommendation to cut back on fat in our diets (rather than to cut back on the *saturated* fat) Americans took it to heart, literally. Americans have made significant cutbacks in dietary fat over the past decades—without any significant decreases in cancer, diabetes, obesity, or coronary heart disease. It appears that we downed all those funny tasting low-fat imitation foods in vain, but why?

First of all, fat is a necessary part of our diets. We cannot live without eating fat. Fat is filling and satisfying. It has great mouth feel and makes things taste good. It is the type of fat, not the amount we eat that makes the difference in our health. Certain types of fats are *good* for us.

*It is the type of fat, not the amount we eat that makes the difference in our health. Certain types of fats are good for us.*

- ∾ The monosaturated fats (found in canola oil, peanut oil, most nuts and peanuts, olives and olive oil, and avocados) and
- ∾ polyunsaturated fats (found in corn oil, soybeans and soybean oil, safflower oil, cottonseed oil, and fish) are beneficial to our bodies.

These "good" fats help our cholesterol profiles by increasing the HDL (the good cholesterol) and decreasing the LDL (the bad cholesterol). This helps protect us from heart attacks and stroke.

Special subtypes of polyunsaturated fats known collectively as *omega-3 fatty acids* are especially good for us. They're called "essential" fatty acids. That means that while they are essential to our body's normal function, we cannot make them ourselves and have to get them from our food. Omega-3 fatty acids help prevent and treat heart disease, help prevent stroke, help prevent sudden death from abnormal heart rhythms, and decrease inflammation.

It's wise to get at least one source of omega-3s in your diet each day. The best source is fish.

## How Can I Get Enough Omega-3 Fatty Acids if I Don't Care for Fish?

If eating fish two to three times a week is not an option, mercury-free fish oil supplements are your best bet. Flaxseeds contain a different type of omega-3 fatty acid, but can also benefit the body. Add *ground* flaxseeds (whole flaxseeds pass through the digestive system undigested) to cereals, baked goods, and salads. (Flaxseeds are easy to grind in a coffee grinder, or they may be purchased ground.) Ground flaxseeds must be kept in the refrigerator and protected from light. They go rancid quickly at room temperature. Flaxseed oil is another option, but goes rancid even more quickly and isn't as tasty as the ground seeds. Eating a daily serving of walnuts or using walnut oil for salads or in baked goods is another option. Canola oil and to a lesser degree soybean oil contain small amounts of omega-3s, so it makes sense to use them as primary sources of fat for salads, cooking, and baking. There is a leafy green Mediterranean vegetable called purslane that is high in omega-3s, but I have yet to see it at the supermarket or even the health food stores. If you can't get your omega-3 fatty acids in your diet, it's a good idea to take fish oil capsules. Make sure that they have been tested and found free of mercury and other contaminants.

## Does that Mean I Can Eat as Much of the Healthy Fats as I Want?

Not exactly. It's true that you can indulge in peanut butter and nuts and enjoy your salad without obsessing about the amount of fat in the salad dressing (as long as it's made with healthy fats), but a word of caution is in order. While the polyunsaturated and monosaturated are indeed good for you, fats contain a lot of calories, more than twice as many calories per gram as sugars and proteins. Consuming more calories than we burn is what makes us fat, period. We need to eat more polyunsaturated and monosaturated fats without eating more calories. That means something else has to go. The simplest thing to do is to *substitute* healthy fats for the unhealthy fats as often as possible.

# Which Fats Do I Need to Avoid?

The unhealthy fats that we want to avoid are the

- ∾ saturated fats (found in meat, animal fat, dairy products, palm oil, and coconut oil) and
- ∾ trans fats (found in margarine, vegetable shortenings, partially hydrogenated vegetable oils, and a plethora of fast foods, commercial baked goods, and snack foods).

These oils not only raise LDL but also lower HDL. The **trans fats** are especially harmful to our bodies. In addition to changing our cholesterol profiles for the worse, trans fats also cause the blood components called platelets to stick together more readily, increasing the likelihood of stroke and heart-attack-causing clots in the blood vessels. The incidence of heart disease in our country increased following the same pattern as the increase in use of trans fats over the past century.

*The incidence of heart disease in our country increased following the same pattern as the increase in use of trans fats over the past century.*

Trans fats are chemicals created in a laboratory that do not exist in nature. They started out as perfectly healthy natural vegetable oils. The oils were treated with a chemical process called partial hydrogenation to deliberately remove the healthy omega-3 fatty acids, which unfortunately cause oils to spoil more rapidly. Since the newly created trans fats had a longer shelf life, they were more desirable to the food industry and became widely distributed throughout our food supply.

# How Can I Avoid Trans Fats?

Unfortunately, manufacturers were not required to disclose the amount of trans fat in a product until January of 2006. Even now, they can tout that their foods have "no trans fat per serving" if the amount in a serving is less than .5 grams. If there is less than .5 grams of trans fat in a food you eat rarely, don't worry about it. If the foods you eat on a regular basis contain trans fats, it's best to switch brands. You still have to read the label to look for the code words that mean trans fat. Avoid any products that contain "shortening" or "partially hydrogenated" oils of any sort.

Sadly, as you start to read labels looking for trans fats, the words "partially hydrogenated" or "shortening" will start popping out at you from most of the labels on the grocery store shelves. They are so thoroughly integrated into our food supply that it's hard to find processed foods without them. Fortunately health food manufacturers, some major snack food companies like Frito-Lay, and some fast food companies like Chick-fil-A are starting to eliminate trans fats from their foods.

*Since the FDA is still allowing food manufacturers to use trans fats, it's up to the individual to look for the code words that mean trans fat. We need to read labels to protect ourselves.*

Read labels and ask restaurants for nutritional information so you can make an informed choice about what you eat. Since the FDA is still allowing food manufacturers to use trans fats, it's up to the individual to look for the code words that mean trans fat. We need to read labels to protect ourselves.

## How Can I Substitute Healthy Fats for Unhealthy Fats in Recipes?

When choosing the fat you want to cook with, bake with, or toss with your salad, it's a little easier. Don't choose fats that are solid at room temperature. Saturated fats like butter and trans fats like margarine are generally solid at room temperature, but healthy fats like canola and olive oils are liquid. Do not buy trans-fat-containing margarine or vegetable shortening.

For sautéing or stir-frying, substitute canola, corn, olive, or peanut oil for butter, margarine, or shortening. Substitute canola oil for butter, lard, or shortening in baking. Use cooking sprays made from olive or canola oil. While substituting healthy oils for the fats traditionally used in baked goods can cause some change in the texture and taste of the final product, fresh homemade baked goods generally taste better than prepackaged goods that contain the trans fats.

You can substitute healthy oils for unhealthy measure for measure. When making substitutions in an old family recipe, you may want to try substituting healthy oil for half of the butter at first, and try substituting a greater percentage next time if you can't tell the difference. (Even Granny might not notice the missing butter in her pound cake.) Baked goods made with canola oil rather than butter tend to be moister. Biscuits and piecrusts will have a less flaky texture when made without trans fats. Butter crusts and biscuits have superior flavor to those made with trans fats; and while butter is not ideal, it's better nutritionally than trans fats.

The only other reason to use butter is if a specific "butter taste" is desired. Even then, the new trans-fat-free butter substitutes or butter-oil blends might suit your palate. If so, they make a much better option than butter on your toast and pancakes.

Nuts and nut oils can often add flavor and nutrition to traditional baked goods. Try nut butters or oils in place of butter on toast and pancakes. Dip bread in olive oil rather than slathering with butter. Olive, canola, corn, or nut oils taste great in salad dressings, and freshly prepared dressings taste infinitely better than the bottled type.

Food should not be deep fat fried, but if you can't do without French fries or other fried foods, make sure they are fried in peanut oil or another healthy oil. The best alternative would be to try one of the recipes in this book for oven roasted "fries."

# Can I Eat Meat and Still Limit Saturated Fats?

It's possible to limit your intake of saturated fats without becoming vegetarian, but it's wise to eat less meat than the average American. Eat vegetable protein sources like nuts and beans as often as possible and substitute fish for red meat at least two times a week. When you do eat beef or pork, eat small portions and limit it to seven, three-ounce portions a week. Less is better. Opt for white meat chicken or turkey prepared without the skin over red meat. Use less fatty cuts of meat and trim the visible fat.

Choose low-fat dairy products like skim milk, low-fat yogurt, or fat-free yogurt. Limit high-fat dairy products like cheese, ice cream, and sour cream. Dairy products are one of the few areas where the low-fat craze did us some good. There are now good tasting low-fat versions of sour cream, cream cheese, yogurt, and even ice cream available, but watch out for added sugar and preservatives.

---

### Savvy Eating Info: The Fats of Life

While we should strive to avoid trans fats altogether, it is not desirable and almost impossible to completely avoid saturated fats. They're found throughout nature. Even the healthy oils that are predominantly monosaturated or polyunsaturated contain some saturated fat. That is part of the reason we can't eat unlimited amounts of healthy oils. Eating less red meat and full-fat dairy products are the most important changes to make when you want to decrease the amount of saturated fat you eat.

---

## *Summary*

Fat is good for us if the right kinds of fats are eaten in moderation. Try to:

1. Avoid trans fats altogether.
2. Reduce the amount of saturated fat in your diet by eating less red meat and fatty dairy products.
3. Eat a source of omega-3 fatty acids like fish, flaxseed, walnuts, or canola oil every day.
4. Don't just add the healthy fats to your diet, **substitute** them for the unhealthy fats you already eat so you do not increase the number of calories you eat.

# CHAPTER 9

# The Skinny on Carbohydrates

Carbohydrates have received a lot of bad press lately from fad diets. Most Americans have heard enough talk from low-carb enthusiasts that they feel a little guilty every time they eat a potato even if they are not sure why. While there's no need to worry about every gram of carbohydrate you put in your mouth, it's important to understand how carbohydrates affect you body. You might even want to forget what you have learned from TV stars and popular magazines for the moment and start over with just the facts on carbs.

## Understanding Glycemic Load

Carbohydrates are a vast group of foods that are predominantly made up of plant sugars and starches. (Lactose, found in milk, is the only non-plant source of carbohydrates.) They provide a readily available energy source, provide almost half of the world's calories, and wield control over our blood sugar.

All carbohydrates provide four calories per gram and cause the hormone insulin to be released when they enter the blood stream, but that's where their similarities end. Carbohydrates include such diverse foods as table sugar (sucrose), potatoes, pasta, apples, oatmeal, beans, and breads.

Some carbohydrate containing foods like beans and oats are full of vital nutrients and fiber. Other carbohydrates like corn syrup, white pasta, and white bread have been stripped of any nutrition and fiber that they had once contained and are basically empty calories. Clearly all carbohydrates are not created equal.

Because carbohydrates exert control over blood sugar, it's vital to your health that you choose your carbohydrates carefully. As described previously, all carbohydrate foods can be assigned a glycemic index (GI). The higher the GI, the faster and more dramatic the effect the food has on the blood sugar. The faster the carbohydrate you eat reaches the blood stream, the more insulin you release. The surge of insulin quickly stores away the carbohydrate you have eaten as fat. Then the blood sugar can drop too fast and too much. This causes you to feel irritable and hungry because the steady supply of glucose your brain needs to function has just been stored away as fat. At this point you usually reach for something else to eat.

A steady diet of high glycemic load (GL) foods causes you to be in a constant cycle of feeling hungry, eating, raising your blood glucose, chasing it with insulin, and storing the glucose as fat only to feel hungry again soon. Because high GL foods cause you to feel hungry sooner than slowly digested low GL carbs, you end up eating more, which generally leads to obesity.

# How Do I Know which Foods Have a Low Glycemic Index?

The GI of a food is actually a number determined in a laboratory on a small group of real people. Currently, there's no standardization of GI values. Different laboratories often get different numbers for the same foods.

While there are lists of the GI value of foods available on the Internet, they're not available on the labels of the foods we buy. Even if those numbers were conveniently available, they're a little difficult to interpret for practical use.

The problem is that the GI is determined for the amount of food that contains fifty grams of carbohydrate. That's about how much carbohydrate is in a cup of white rice. You might realistically eat a one-cup serving of rice, so the GI of forty-five would give you some idea of the impact of that food on your blood sugar.

But let's say you want to eat a carrot. Carrots have a whopping GI of 131! Do carrots really have that dramatic effect on your blood sugar? Well, the answer is yes if you eat about a pound and a half of them, because that is how much you would have to eat to get fifty grams of carbohydrate. However, a half-cup serving of carrots, which contains about ten grams of carbohydrate, would have about one-fifth the impact on your blood sugar that a fifty-gram serving would have. This is why the concept of "glycemic load" was developed.

*The glycemic load (GL) is the impact that a single serving of a food will have on your blood sugar*

The glycemic load (GL) is the impact that a single serving of a food will have on your blood sugar.

The GL of ¾ cup of white rice is thirty-four, and the GL of ½ cup of carrots is eleven. Therefore, a serving of carrots has a lower GL and less impact on your blood sugar than a serving of refined white rice.

While the glycemic load gives us a more accurate picture of how a food will impact our blood sugar, determining a food's glycemic load is complicated. So we need some guidelines to determine the relative glycemic load of the foods we eat without cumbersome charts and calculations.

In general, carbohydrate-containing foods can be divided into four categories: low GL, moderate GL, high GL, and very high GL (empty carbs).

- ∾ Most vegetables, legumes, citrus fruits, and berries have a *low GL*, and have lots of other good reasons to eat them, so you can enjoy them with impunity.
- ∾ All other fruits (except for dried fruits and tropical fruits like mangoes, pineapples, and bananas) have *moderate GL* and should be eaten in moderation (no more than three servings a day).
- ∾ Whole grains (including brown rice, oats, and stone ground whole wheat) and natural starches (including potatoes and whole-grain pasta), and sweet fruits (including dried fruits, fruit juices, and tropical fruit) have a *high GL* and should be eaten in small portions. (See chapter 12 for a chart of portion sizes.) These foods do have a significant impact on your blood sugar, but they also have health benefits from antioxidants, fiber, and healthy fats. They're an important part of a healthy diet.
- ∾ Refined grains (like white bread, white pasta, crackers, pretzels, and chips), sweets (like graham crackers, cookies, cakes, sweet cereals, most breakfast bars, and candy) and sweetened beverages have *very high GL* and very little nutritional merit, so they're empty carbs that should be avoided.

## Why Should I Eat Whole Grains?

Whole grains are a great source of many nutrients and are very satisfying. They also make a complete protein when combined with legumes and are a vital part of vegetarian diets. It's necessary to eat grains whole and unprocessed because most of the nutrients found in them are destroyed when the grain is refined.

When the outer bran layer of the grain is removed, 78 percent of the fiber, 85 percent of the magnesium, and most of the vitamins are lost. When the inner germ layer is removed, we lose 95 percent of the vitamin E and most of the healthy oils. Whole grains contain vitamins, minerals, healthy fats, and other micronutrients that work together to prevent disease and nourish our bodies. Fortification of refined grains does not replace all the nutrients that processing strips from the whole grains.

Eating whole grains along with the fiber they naturally contain is crucial. Fiber slows the digestion of the whole grain lowering the GL. Adding fiber to your diet in the form of a pill has never been shown to have any health benefits other than decreasing constipation. In order to get the cancer, heart disease, and stroke-fighting benefits of whole grains, you need to eat the grains intact.

Because grains have a large amount of carbohydrate per serving, they have a significant impact on blood sugar. However, whole grains like brown rice, old-fashioned oats, and cracked wheat have a lower GL than their processed counterparts—white rice, processed sweetened instant oatmeal, and finely ground flour. It's important to eat grains that are *unprocessed* as well as *whole*.

## How Can I Tell which Foods Are Whole Grain?

Thanks to dishonest food labeling, that isn't as easy as it should be. Often "wheat" breads and "multigrain" breads contain very little whole grain. "Brown bread" or "honey wheat bread," which is often made with highly refined whole-wheat flour, can have a GL similar to white bread if the flour is very finely ground. The less processed a grain, the lower its GL. Look for breads with visible variation in texture, nuts, seeds, or large pieces of grains.

Some cereal manufacturers have launched campaigns that advertise more whole grains in their cereals. While adding more whole grains is a good thing, the labeling of these foods is tricky. "Made with whole grain" does not mean that it's a whole grain cereal. The cereal might be made of white rice, refined corn, or cornstarch with a little whole wheat or oats thrown in. Ingredients like white rice flour, corn meal, and cornstarch have a very high GL.

> *"Made with whole grain" does not mean that it's a whole grain cereal.*

Make sure that the first ingredient in your bread or cereal is whole grain: whole-wheat flour, brown rice, whole oats, or another whole grain. In general, whole-grain breads and cereals will contain about three grams of fiber for every one hundred calories. If it contains significantly less fiber, it's probably not whole grain.

> *In general, whole-grain breads and cereals will contain about three grams of fiber for every one hundred calories.*

I suggest you try a variety of whole grains: quinoa, barley, brown rice, whole-grain pastas, wheat berries, oats, and kasha. Try these new grains instead of white rice, potatoes, or white pasta.

Several brands of whole-wheat and brown-rice pasta are now available in large grocery stores. Brown rice adds a whole new dimension to

## Savvy Eating Info: How Processing Grains Affects the Nutritive Value of Whole Grains

Whole-grain unprocessed oats are little rounded grains like grains of rice. They take about half an hour to cook, longer to digest, and have a relatively low GL. Old-fashioned oats are whole oats that have been squashed flat. They cook in about five minutes, and have a greater surface area, enabling digestive enzymes to break them down faster, yielding a somewhat higher GL. Instant oatmeals are oats that are squashed flat then ground up into small bits. These small bits cook in less than a minute and have a lot of surface area, which speeds digestion. Therefore, they have a higher GL. All three types of oats are whole grains. They have the same nutrients, the same amount of fiber, and the same number of calories, but have different effects on the body because of the way they are processed. The unprocessed oats will fill you up longer than the other types, even though they have the same number of calories. Unprocessed foods have less impact on your blood sugar and are better for you.

How the grain is cooked also affects the GL. Pasta cooked to al dente or still a little chewy, has a moderately high GL. Overcooked pasta, which is waterlogged and mushy, has a higher GL. Both pastas are similar nutritionally, but their effects on blood sugar are different because the mushy pasta is digested more rapidly.

*Do I have to subsist on chewy undercooked whole grains?*

No. While unprocessed and chewy whole grains have the gentlest effect on your blood sugar, palatability is very important. For some, the chewy wholesome unprocessed oat is worth waiting thirty minutes for in the morning. For me, I would rather microwave my old-fashioned oats for three minutes and enjoy them with a little maple syrup and fruit, even though my version has a higher GL. It's worth it to me for the palatability and convenience. They still satisfy me until noon. Everyone must find his or her happy medium.

pilafs. The hearty flavor and texture stands up to exotic flavors and is amazingly filling. If you have tried brown rice before and did not care for it, be sure to try a quality brand like Lundberg's. Delicious filling pilafs can be made with a variety of whole grains, each with their own unique taste and texture. Quick-cooking barley that is ready in less time than it takes to cook white rice is now available. Like oats, barley has a dramatic effect on lowering cholesterol. Try as many different whole grains as you can; you may find a new favorite.

When baking, replace half or more of the white flour called for in a recipe with whole-wheat flour. If you find whole wheat a little heavy for some baked goods, try using sorghum flour instead (look for it at health food stores). Soy flower can replace ¼- to ½-cup flour in most recipes and add protein as well as fiber.

# Do Proteins and Fats Affect Blood Sugar?

Proteins and fats themselves do not have much effect on blood sugar or insulin release. However, fats and proteins do slow digestion and can thereby decrease a carbohydrate-containing food's GL. For example, a 200-calorie bowl of oatmeal made with milk has a lower GL than a 200-calorie bowl of oatmeal made with water, because the protein in the milk slows the digestion of the oatmeal's carbohydrates. This is part of the reason that the "low-fat" refined carbohydrate snacks that became popular over the past twenty years have been so harmful to our health. Cookies and crackers are empty calories with high GL to begin with, but taking out the fat boosts the GL even higher.

# What Harm Do High GL Foods Cause?

With a diet of predominantly high GL foods, the body is forced to produce much larger amounts of insulin to control the amount of sugar being dumped into the blood stream. The blood sugar drops fast and sometimes too low. Low blood sugar makes you grouchy and hungry, so you eat more. This glycemic roller coaster is a leading cause of obesity. Obese people are more likely to develop type 2 diabetes.

For reasons that are not entirely known, the body can become "insulin resistant." That means that insulin no longer enables the body's cells to take in glucose the way they should. In turn, more and more insulin is produced, yet the blood sugar remains dangerously elevated. This condition is called type 2 diabetes. The body keeps producing insulin, but the blood sugar continues to rise because the body's cells have decreased ability to take in glucose. They become resistant to insulin.

Over time, the overworked insulin-producing cells in your pancreas can just wear out, and your body is no longer able to produce the insulin needed to make use of the sugar your digestive system has deposited in your blood. Type 2 diabetes starts as just insulin resistance, but it generally becomes a combination of insulin resistance and overworked, inadequate insulin-producing cells.

Certainly genes play a role in determining how much abuse from high

GL foods your system can take. Other players include obesity, inactivity, and a higher body fat to muscle tissue ratio. Some people develop diabetes relatively early in life even if they don't always eat high GL foods. Others can subsist primarily on refined high GL foods and not develop diabetes if they lived one hundred years. Those people are rare. Diabetes is the number six killer in the United States.

Diabetes is more common in some cultures than others. Industrialized nations tend to have the highest rates of diabetes. The incidence of diabetes is inversely proportional to the amount of regular physical activity a population gets. Those who get more exercise have more lean muscle tissue and less fat. These people tend not to be obese and tend not to have diabetes.

> *The incidence of diabetes is inversely proportional to the amount of regular physical activity a population gets.*

## Can I Eat Too Many Carbohydrates?

Yes. Because of the convenience, availability, and most people's taste preferences for sweets and grain products, our society has become overly dependent on them as a major source of calories. Nutritionally empty carbohydrates like soft drinks, cakes, cookies, quick breads, doughnuts, sugars, syrups, jams, and white potatoes account for over a quarter of our daily calories. Eating too many carbohydrates is a major culprit in today's epidemic of obesity and chronic disease.

However, if you get the majority of your carbohydrates from vegetables, citrus fruits, and berries, it's very unlikely that you could eat too many carbohydrates. Grains are another story. While you should include whole grains and fruits in you diet because of the many nutrients that they contain that help ward off cancer and other diseases, it is possible to overeat these carbohydrates. Don't eat huge portions of carbohydrates.

Aim for one to three portions per meal (like a sandwich made with two slices of bread and an apple), not the four to six portions contained in an average fast-food meal (breaded chicken on a deli roll and a regular order of fries). Even nutritious foods like whole grains and fruits *eaten in excess* are detrimental to your health. Moderation is key.

Empty carbs should be avoided as much as possible because even small portions have a high GL. All carbohydrates cause insulin release. And insulin's darker side causes storage of fat, increased blood pressure, increased LDL, and increased incidence of heart attack and stroke. While releasing some insulin is necessary and normal, causing huge fluctuations in blood sugar and insulin by eating large portions of carbohydrates, especially high GL carbs is unhealthy.

### Savvy Eating Info: The Many Roles of Insulin

Insulin is one of the body's most important hormones. While it's usually known for its effect on blood sugar, it actually has many vital roles. The roles of insulin include:

- lowering elevated blood sugar
- converting glucose and protein to fat
- converting dietary fat to fat stored in our body's fat cells
- increasing the body's production of cholesterol
- stimulating the growth of arterial smooth muscle cells
- making the kidneys hold on to excess fluids

That's a lot of functions for one hormone, and the carbohydrates that we eat affect all of insulin's functions. When we eat more carb calories than we need, our efficient little hormone, insulin, rushes into the blood stream and neatly stores all our excess calories as fat.

This leads to excess poundage, but that's not all. As we stimulate our bodies to produce more insulin by overeating, we increase our LDL (the bad cholesterol), making us more likely to have a heart attack or stroke. It doesn't stop there. It also causes the smooth muscle cells in our arteries to bulk up, making heart attacks and strokes even more likely. Then insulin causes the kidneys to retain fluid. This causes our blood pressure to go up—a triple whammy for heart attacks and strokes. That is part of the reason why cultures like our own, which base diets on lots of refined carbohydrates, tend to have more obesity, diabetes, high-blood pressure, heart attacks, and strokes.

The amount of insulin we produce eating a low GL diet or the amount of insulin a diabetic needs to regulate blood sugar is unlikely to cause problems. However, eating a high GL diet can cause side effects from insulin's darker side.

**The bottom line is when you eat carbohydrates, you want to choose ones with a low GL so you are satisfied with less and keep your blood sugar steady. The more steady your blood sugar, the better.**

It is of critical importance that diabetics who are prescribed insulin take it as directed by their doctor. While a high GL diet and excess insulin is harmful, the sustained high blood sugar that an insulin dependent diabetic would experience without taking insulin is much worse and could be deadly in a short period of time. Insulin dependent diabetics need their insulin, but benefit from a low GL diet.

*In general, if you maintain a healthy body weight, limiting your intake of very high GL foods (empty carbs) to two or fewer per day is a reasonable goal.*

In general, if you maintain a healthy body weight, limiting your intake of very high GL foods (*empty* carbs) to two or fewer per day is a reasonable goal. (Remember that beverages like sweet wine, beer, sodas, sweetened fruit drinks, and sweetened tea, as well as white bread, pretzels, crackers, and white pasta fall into the empty carb category.) If you're trying to lose weight, try to limit **empty** carbs to no more than one serving a day. Most children and those who exercise regularly can consume more without harm.

Limit how many moderate to high GL carbohydrates (fruits, whole grains, and starchy vegetables) you eat at one time. Don't eat bread, a baked potato, sweetened apple sauce, and cookies all in the same meal. It's fine to eat healthy carbohydrates throughout the day, but don't eat a lot of them at a single meal or snack. Active adults and children do not need to limit their moderate and high GL carbohydrate intake as long as they maintain a healthy weight and spread their carbohydrates out over the day.

Eat as many low GL carbohydrates (vegetables, citrus fruits, and berries) as you care to eat. Most of your servings of carbohydrates should be vegetables, fruits, or whole grains.

The following chart lists various carbohydrate foods in terms of

- ∾ *Green-light carbs:* vegetables, citrus fruits, and berries with *low GL*
- ∾ *Yellow-light carbs:* nutritious foods with *moderate to high GL*
- ∾ *Red-light carbs: very high GL* carbs with little nutritional value.

Eat green-light carbs often. Eat yellow-light carbs in moderation. These are good healthy foods, but they do have a significant glycemic effect. Eat no more than three servings from this category per meal or limit portion size. For example, rather than eating a large serving of pasta and a whole-wheat roll, choose either bread *or* pasta for that meal, or simply eat smaller portions of both. Avoid red-light carbs as much as possible.

### Savvy Eating Info: Types of GL Carbs

| Green-light (Low GL) | Yellow-light (Moderate GL) | Yellow-light (High GL) | Red-light (Very High GL) |
|---|---|---|---|
| *Enjoy as many as you care to eat.* | *Nutritious foods with moderate GL. Don't hesitate to include these foods in your diet, they contain many nutrients. Just eat small portions in moderation.* | *Nutritious foods with high GL. Don't hesitate to include these foods in your diet, they contain many nutrients. Just eat small portions in moderation.* | *Empty carbs. Avoid or limit to one or two a day.* |
| **Berries:** strawberries, raspberries, blueberries, cranberries, etc. | **Most fruits:** Apples, pears, peaches, grapes, plums, melons, cherries, nectarines | 100% fruit juice, bananas, raisins, mango, pineapple, prunes, dates, figs, dried apricots, and other dried fruits, etc. | **Refined-grain products:** white rice, white bread, white rolls and buns, snack crackers, pretzels, corn chips, graham crackers, white pasta, cakes, cookies, refined-grain muffins, most power and granola bars, pop tarts, bagels, biscuits, etc." |
| **Citrus fruits:** oranges, grapefruit, etc. | | **Whole grains:** Brown rice, stone-ground whole wheat, quinoa, rye, oats, barley, corn, whole-grain breads etc. | **Beverages:** beer, sweet wine, sweet tea, sweetened soft drinks, fruit drinks |
| **Other fruits:** avocado, olives | | **Starches:** whole-grain pasta, white potatoes, sweet potato, etc | |
| **Most vegetables:** peas, beans, lentils, spinach, lettuce and other greens, carrots, squash, asparagus, broccoli, cabbage, onions, peppers, herbs, pumpkin, turnips, garlic, etc. | | | |

# Are High Carbohydrate Diets Harmful?

For most people, yes. While some people, about one-fourth of the population, are genetically programmed to tolerate a diet high in carbs and yet remain thin, maintain normal blood pressure, and low LDL cholesterol, for most of us, a high carb diet spells trouble. High-carbohydrate,

> ## Savvy Eating Tips: Cutting Down on Carbs Can Make Weight Loss Easier
>
> If you're overweight, next to exercising, cutting down the amount of carbohydrates, especially refined carbohydrates and sweet drinks, is the single most effective way to lose weight. Limit your empty carbs to one a day, and your yellow-light carbs to four to five servings a day, five to six if you're exercising most days. Do this by substituting green-light fruits and vegetables for some of your yellow- and red-light foods.
>
> - Choose water over a sweet drink or juice
> - Choose oranges or strawberries over bananas or raisins
> - Choose whole-grain pasta over white
> - Eat a smaller portion of pasta with a larger portion of veggies
> - Choose green beans over French fries
>
> These small changes can add up to big differences on the scale.

low-fat diets have been linked with increased incidence of heart disease, stroke, and diabetes.

Lean active adults and children tolerate a diet high in carbohydrates better than their sedentary obese counterparts. People with excess fat and low muscle mass are particularly susceptible to the negative effects of insulin. That explains, in part, how skinny teenagers can down cokes and fries on a daily basis without gaining a pound. Age will catch up with them eventually, and the ravages of the high GL diet will set in.

If you eat like most Americans, you may need to make drastic changes in your carbohydrate intake. If you're overweight or sedentary, you need to limit the amount of carbohydrates you consume and make sure that the carbohydrates you do eat are vegetables, fruits, and unrefined-whole grains. If the breads, cakes, cookies, bagels, buns, rolls, and other refined carbohydrates you consume on a daily basis aren't the absolute tastiest things you eat, don't eat them! Simply leave out the plain white bun that comes with your burger, or the crackers that came with the salad. Life is too short for mediocre bread! On the other hand, if you look forward to the glass of wine or the chocolate cake you plan to have at the end of the day, enjoy it. But limit your indulgences to a couple a day.

If you find yourself dozing off or needing caffeine about two to three hours after a meal, chances are your meal was too high in carbohydrates. Cut back on your carbohydrates and increase the protein you eat until you no longer get sleepy or irritable two to three hours after a meal or snack.

---

**Savvy Eating Tip: If You Want to Eat a Lot of Carbs,
You Need to Be Active**

That means doing vigorous activity for forty-five to sixty minutes most days of the week. If you choose not to be physically active on a regular basis, you cannot afford to eat large amounts of carbohydrates without significantly increasing your chances of obesity, stroke, heart disease, and diabetes.

---

# What about Artificial Sweeteners?

That's a good question. Nobody really knows whether consuming artificial sweeteners on a regular basis causes cancer many years down the road. Unless you're diabetic, you may want to avoid artificial sweeteners just in case. Artificial sweeteners are very useful for diabetics to use on a regular basis and are fine for occasional use for most people. However, if you're using an artificial sweetener more than twice a week, you may want to find substitutes for those foods. Drink water rather than soda, sweeten yogurt with a small amount of honey (which has a lower GL than sugar), drink your coffee without sweetener or opt for a small amount of sugar.

*It's better to develop a taste for less sweet foods by gradually decreasing the amount of sugar in your diet than encouraging your taste for sweets with artificial sweeteners.*

It's better to develop a taste for less sweet foods by gradually decreasing the amount of sugar in your diet than encouraging your taste for sweets with artificial sweeteners. (Replace some of the sweets in your diet with some of the lower-sugar recipes in this book.) The less sugar you eat, the less you will crave.

---

## Summary

1. Eat plenty of vegetables, citrus fruits, and berries without worrying about the number of carbohydrates or their glycemic effect.
2. Choose whole-grain breads, cereals, cooked grains, and pastas over refined ones because of the fiber and micronutrients they contain.
3. Choose less-processed, rough-textured whole grains whenever possible.

4. Limit very high GL carbohydrates (including sweet beverages, sweets, white bread, white pasta, or refined grains) to two or less a day most days.

5. If you need to lose weight, eat plenty of green-light carbs, but limit your yellow-light carb intake (that includes some fruits, potatoes, and grains) to four to five servings a day, five to six servings if you're exercising. If you want to eat carbs, you need to exercise.

# CHAPTER 10

# Grandma Was Right:
# Eat Your Fruits and Veggies

Eating a variety of fruits and vegetables is the foundation of a healthy diet. Plant foods contain hundreds of chemicals called phytonutrients that help the body ward off disease. For example:

- Daily consumption of fruits, vegetables, and especially garlic has been associated with decreased risk of death from heart disease and stroke as well as enhanced immune function.
- Cruciferous vegetables like cabbage and broccoli contain iso-thiocyanates and sulforaphane, powerful cancer-fighting compounds.
- Tomatoes contain lycopene, a phytonutrient that helps prevent prostate cancer.
- Beta-carotene in carrots and leafy greens, anthocyanins in colorful berries, organosulfates in garlic and onions, and flavinoids in citrus fruits all help us fight off cancers.

There is no doubt that plant foods are essential to good health. You won't find many people who are unaware that they need to be eating fruits and vegetables, yet Americans eat three or fewer servings of them a day. What are they waiting for?

## What about a Pill with All those Disease-Fighting Phytonutrients?

In our fast-paced society many people prefer a quick fix, like a vitamin pill, to lifestyle changes. *No such pill exists.* Even if there were a pill big enough to contain all the phytonutrients you need for optimal health, it would be more difficult to swallow than the current dietary recommendation of at least five to nine servings of fruits and vegetables a day. In order to get all the disease-fighting benefits of fruits and vegetables, you actually have to eat them.

Many phytonutrients only benefit the body when they're eaten as a whole food. For example, studies have shown that diets high in fruits and vegetables can decrease your chances of developing certain types of cancers. Vitamin A has been shown to slow the development of cancers in lab animals. Vitamin A precursors, called caritenoids, are contained in abundance in many vegetables. Scientists isolated the caritenoids and put them in pill form and studied their effect on cancer.

> Many phytonutrients only benefit the body when they're eaten as a whole food.

Disappointingly, the caritenoids by themselves did not decrease the incidence of cancers. In fact, it appears that the caritenoids might have *increased* the study population's chances of dying of lung cancer. Other studies showed an increase in lung, prostate, and stomach cancer when subjects were treated with large doses of vitamin A alone. However, those who ate a *diet* high in vitamin A showed a decreased incidence of many types of cancer.

We don't know whether there is a substance or group of substances in the whole food that changes the way vitamin A affects the body, or if the anti-cancer effect of these plant foods is due to another as yet undiscovered phytonutrient. It's also not clear how much of a given nutrient is enough or how much is too much. For example, vitamin A is toxic to the liver if too much is taken in pill form, yet it's vital for normal vision, immune function, and cancer prevention.

We *do* know that supplementing the diet with the doses of vitamins within the U.S. recommended daily allowance (USRDA) is safe as well as wise. But the doses found in mega supplements and used in some clinical studies may not be safe. Overdosage of vitamin A, or any other vitamin from foods alone, would be difficult if not impossible. The only proven and safe way to decrease your overall disease risk is to eat a variety of fruits and vegetables daily.

> The only proven and safe way to decrease your overall disease risk is to eat a variety of fruits and vegetables daily.

## How Much Produce Do I Need to Eat?

You need at least five to nine servings a day. What's more, if you're a large person, very active, or have a specific disease prevention goal in mind, the minimum five servings a day is probably not enough. You should aim for the seven to nine range *or more*. The more calories you consume, the more fruits and vegetables you need to eat.

# How Much Is a Serving of
# Fruits and Vegetables?

Use the following chart to find the serving size of various fruits and vegetables. The serving size of some of the fruits and vegetables may be much more or less than you thought. For example, a quarter-cup serving of dried fruit fills the palm of your cupped hand. A half-cup serving of beans fills a small burrito. One cup of cantaloupe fills your cereal bowl. A cup of lettuce covers a small plate, and so on. Get used to how a serving looks on your own dishes as well as in your most frequented restaurants.

### Savvy Eating Info: Serving Sizes

| Type of food | | Serving size |
| --- | --- | --- |
| **Fruits (include at least two to three)** | Melons, and other large fruits, cut up | 1 cup |
| | Apples, pears, oranges, peaches, and other medium-sized fruits | 1 medium-sized whole fruit |
| | Grapes and berries | ½ cup |
| | Dried fruits | ¼ cup |
| | Fruit and vegetable juices | ¾ cup (6 ounces) |
| **Vegetables (include at least three to six)** | Leafy green, raw | 1 cup loosely packed |
| | Other raw vegetables | ½ cup |
| | Cooked, including beans | ½ cup |

# Do All Fruits and Vegetables Benefit
# Your Body Equally Well?

Simply put, no. While most fruits and vegetables do have some health benefits, many are endowed with more disease-fighting power than others. Vegetables tend to have the most benefits, with two major exceptions: white potatoes and iceberg lettuce. These American fast-food staples are sadly lacking in health benefits. Potatoes do contain a number of vitamins and minerals if eaten with the skin, but are mostly made of large quantities of an easily digested starch that causes the blood sugar to soar. Iceberg lettuce is mostly water and pales in comparison to its more colorful relatives like romaine and leaf lettuces in its vitamin content. That doesn't mean that you should never eat these vegetables,

*French fries and potato chips don't count as a vegetable.*

but rather opt for more colorful, more densely nutritious fruits and vegetables when you can. Remember, French fries and potato chips don't count as a vegetable.

## How Do You Know Which Fruits and Vegetables Are the Best for You?

Luckily, you don't need to be a biologist to determine which plant foods you need to be eating. It's nice to know all the names and sources of the phytonutrients discussed in the first paragraph of this chapter, but ultimately unnecessary. Nature has done an awesome job of color-coding plant foods. If you choose a variety of intensely colored fruits and vegetables every day, you will most likely get all the phytonutrients you need. In addition, taking a vitamin with the USRDA of most vitamins is good insurance.

*If you choose a variety of intensely colored fruits and vegetables every day, you will most likely get all the phytonutrients you need.*

## How Can I Fit in Five to Nine Servings of Fruits and Vegetables a Day?

For those of you who are used to three or fewer servings of fruits and vegetables a day, five to nine servings may seem like a challenging if not impossible goal. Eating a variety of plant foods every day can be accomplished with a little planning up front. It would be difficult indeed to eat five (much less nine or more) servings of fruits and vegetables a day if you waited, as many of us do, until supper to fit them all in. That would be one monstrous salad! Making a habit of eating fruits and vegetables throughout the day is the simplest way to get your five to nine a day.

Most people don't care for vegetables first thing in the morning with the occasional exception of a weekend veggie omelet. (I would not count the French fry's close cousin, the hash brown, as a serving of vegetables unless they are made with skin-on potatoes and lots of peppers and onions.)

Breakfast is a good time to enjoy whole grain cereals and fruit. Plan to get a serving or two of fruit each morning and start the day off ahead. Whole fruit in its natural state is the best choice, but if convenience is a big factor, fruit juices are the next best thing. Opt for 100 percent juice purees that are deeply colored for the best nutrition. Purees retain some of the fiber contained in the whole fruit, but watch out for added sugars

*Savvy Eating Info: Superfoods*

There are some fruits and vegetables that are so good for you that it's reasonable to try to include them in your diet every day.

- **Cruciferous vegetables** (kale, broccoli, cauliflower, mustard greens, turnips, collard greens, cabbage, Brussels sprouts, watercress, and others) are cancer-fighting powerhouses.
- **Green leafy vegetables** (spinach, lettuce, collard greens, kale, mustard greens, etc.) contain calcium, magnesium, and vitamin K along with a host of phytonutrients.
- **Legumes** (beans, peas, soybeans, etc.) contain folate and many other cancer- and heart-disease-fighting substances as well as lots of fiber. They're the masters of satiety in the vegetable world. They also serve double duty as a vegetable and a protein source when combined with grains.
- **The onion family** (asparagus, leeks, garlic, shallots, chives, etc.) Contain compounds that both fight cardiovascular disease and cancer.
- **Citrus fruits** (oranges, grapefruit, lemons, limes, and clementines, etc.) are packed with disease-fighting phytochemicals like limonene, vitamin C, and folate.
- **Berries and grapes** contain a host of cancer-fighting substances that often give them their color.

that may be hidden in them. Commercial fruit smoothies are notorious for added sugar; make sure yours is just fruit. Added sugars are nothing more than empty calories. Sugars may be listed on the label as sugar (beet, brown, cane, corn, or other), corn sweetener, corn syrup, dextrin, fructose, galactose, glucose, high fructose corn syrup, honey, lactose, levulose, maltose, mannitol, maple syrup, molasses, sorbitol, or sucrose.

If a whole piece of fruit is too much for you to tackle at breakfast time, consider slicing fruit the night before (or as your coffee brews). Dried fruits like raisins, dates, cranberries, etc., are a simple addition to a bowl of cereal. Frozen raspberries or blueberries can be added to oatmeal before microwave cooking for approximately three minutes for a tasty nutritious treat any time of year.

Snack time is a great time to get in more fruits and veggies. The most obvious way to do this is to snack on raw fruits and vegetables. Dried fruits, whole fresh fruits, and raw veggies make great portable, nutritious snacks. Of course, not everyone likes to munch on a bag of crisp carrot sticks for a snack; but if you do, more power to you. If rabbit food is *not* your bag, it's time to start thinking out of the box. Whoever said that "snack foods" have to be different from the foods we enjoy at meal times? (Perhaps the snack food companies?) If you can't wait to eat the pita with hummus, or veggie sandwich, or bean burrito, or salad, or soup you're having for lunch, don't wait. Parcel out your meals into mini-meals: soup at eleven, salad at one.

*If you can't wait to eat the pita with hummus, or veggie sandwich, or bean burrito, or salad, or soup you're having for lunch, don't wait. Parcel out your meals into mini-meals: soup at eleven, salad at one.*

One of the single most effective ways to eat more fruits and vegetables is to get into the habit of eating them for lunch. One of the simplest ways to get in lunchtime veggies is to plan on eating leftovers for lunch. If this is neither possible nor appealing, go on the soup or salad plan.

Having soup or salad for lunch most days will almost ensure that you get the needed five to nine a day. That said, be sure to choose soups and salads whose main ingredients are fruits and vegetables. For example, canned chicken noodle, clam chowder, or even some brands of cream of broccoli soups might have trace amounts of vegetables in them, but they're mostly salt water with or without full-fat cream and other undesirable ingredients. Choose prepackaged soups with vegetables listed at the top of the label, go to a quality restaurant, or make your own from recipes in this book.

*Having soup or salad for lunch most days will almost ensure that you get the needed five to nine a day. That said, be sure to choose soups and salads whose main ingredients are fruits and vegetables.*

By the same token, if your salad is a mixture of iceberg lettuce, a few pale out of season tomatoes, cheese, and luncheon meats or fried chicken fingers, you probably are not getting a serving of vegetables from your salad. A healthy salad should have a large amount of intensely colored fruits and vegetables in addition to any proteins, dairy products, or other salad toppings.

Suppertime is the classic time to enjoy vegetables. Still, many families only prepare one or two vegetables at the nighttime meal. Frequently, one of the vegetables is the white potato, which is more of a starch than a vegetable. Corn is another popular choice, but it's a grain, not a vegetable. Strive to eat the fruits and vegetables listed in the chart above that give you the most phytonutrients for your money rather than the less nutritious American staples.

Serving fruit as an appetizer or dessert is an enjoyable way to start or finish a meal. Having fruit before a meal is a great technique for losing weight. The water and fiber help fill you up so you become satisfied earlier in the meal and can better resist second helpings or dessert.

It's important to learn time- and effort-saving techniques that make fruit and especially vegetable preparation easy and convenient. Most people don't have the time or desire to be in the kitchen all day. Learning several preparation techniques that can be applied to many different vegetables can help you enjoy a variety of vegetables no matter what is in season.

> *It's important to learn time- and effort-saving techniques that make fruit and especially vegetable preparation easy and convenient.*

For example, as you will see in the chapter on roasting, the same roasting technique can be applied to sweet potatoes, Brussels sprouts, squash, and onions, as well as proteins like chicken or fish. You can easily prepare a bountiful and varied meal with very little effort or mess. Once you learn a technique, you can create variety by interchanging spice blends and using different vegetables. One-pot veggie and pasta dishes are quick to prepare, but never boring because the variety of vegetables and sauces that can be used is endless. For others developing a repertoire of easy prep dishes that can be prepared in advance and frozen is the answer. All of these techniques and more are explained later in this book. Once you have figured out what works for you, Savvy Eating becomes habit.

## Does It Matter How I Prepare My Vegetables?

Yes. Boiling vegetables depletes them of many nutrients that are watersoluble. You can actually see the water change color as the vegetable cooks creating a vegetable broth. Unless you plan to use the broth for soup, another preparation method will yield better nutrition.

Steamed vegetables lose less of their nutrients, but still lose some. Roasting and stir-frying cause very little loss of nutrients. Eating your vegetables raw is an excellent option, but some have difficulty digesting large amounts of raw vegetables. Some vegetables like carrots and tomatoes actually become more nutritious when cooked. It's difficult for us to

> *Roasting and stir-frying cause very little loss of nutrients.*

break down the cell walls in raw carrots. Cooking the carrots causes the cell walls to break down so we can more readily use the phytonutrients in them. Likewise, cooking tomatoes concentrates the lycopene they contain. Eating lots of fruits and vegetables is the goal no matter what preparation method you choose. When it comes to getting more veggies

*When it comes to getting more veggies into your diet, the most important issues are ease of preparation and great taste.*

into your diet, the most important issues are ease of preparation and great taste.

No matter how nutritious vegetables are, most people won't get enough if they don't taste good, or if they're extremely difficult to prepare. If you grew up on southern-style soul food and collards just aren't worth eating cooked without salt pork, then by all means eat them that way. It's probably more important to get the vegetables into your diet than to worry about the seasonings. (Be sure to use nitrite-free pork.) However, most good old-fashioned recipes can be modified to be more healthful without sacrificing taste. You can often cut back on the amount of salt and saturated fat by half without making a major change in the taste.

*Most good old-fashioned recipes can be modified to be more healthful without sacrificing taste.*

Fruits on the other hand are best eaten raw and unprocessed. While applesauce, peach smoothies, and blueberry cobblers rank high on most people's favorite food lists, they tend to contain lots of undesirable added sugars or trans or saturated fats. Reach for raw fruits most of the time and save the fruit recipes for treats.

## Does It Matter Whether I Buy Organic Produce?

Yes, but nobody knows *how much* it matters. Organic produce has been shown to have dramatically less pesticide residue than conventionally grown produce.

Do the pesticide residues found on conventional produce cause harm? If so, how much does it take to cause health problems? These questions have not yet been answered. Until we know more, it is prudent to eat organic produce whenever it is available and affordable.

*If you often eat apples, carrots, celery, grapes or raisins, green beans, lettuce, oranges, peaches, peanuts, potatoes, strawberries, or wheat, you may want to look for organic sources.*

Some fruits and vegetables are found to be more heavily pesticide contaminated than others. If you often eat apples, carrots, celery, grapes or raisins, green beans, lettuce, oranges, peaches, peanuts, potatoes, strawberries, or wheat, you may want to look for organic sources.

Organic produce has another advantage over conventional produce. Organic fruits and vegetables can actually contain more antioxidants than produce treated with pesticides. In theory, the organic plants produce the antioxidants to protect themselves from pests. So it makes sense to buy organic produce for food safety and a health benefit reasons as well as for ecological reasons.

## How Am I Going to Feel after I Eat All These Fruits and Vegetables?

For the most part, great! However, most people who dramatically increase their fruit and vegetable consumption over a short period of time experience a few side effects. (For those of you whose disposition is too delicate to discuss flatulence you may skip this paragraph, but I recommend you read it.) A large part of the fruits and vegetables we eat are actually indigestible. From a health perspective, that's a good thing. The indigestible parts, such as fiber, slow digestion, reduce the insulin response, increase satiety, and help regulate the colon, preventing constipation and helping us rid the body of unwanted substances like excess cholesterol.

However, people have varying degrees of abilities to absorb natural sugars contained in plant foods. If these sugars remain in the gut, they ferment and form methane and hydrogen gas, the source of flatulence, bloating, and discomfort. Thus a diet high in healthy fruits and vegetables can have some unpleasant side effects.

Back in the days of working on the farm, this was not a big deal. However, in the modern age of the business meeting and the office cubicle, it can be a significant problem. To avoid excessive flatulence, add more fruits and vegetables to the diet slowly over several weeks. Start out with most of the additions to your diet being cooked rather than raw, and go for smaller more frequent servings.

Many people have some degree of fructose (a sugar found in most fruits) intolerance. It will help to eat small servings of fruit at a time. Many benefit from eating their fruits at a separate time from other foods because we digest fruits somewhat differently than other foods.

Eventually, almost everyone adjusts to the high-produce diet. If painful gas and bloating persist after the first few weeks, you may be constipated. (Constipation means hard or lumpy stools no matter what the frequency. Constipation impairs escape of gas from the colon causing painful gas build up.) If you have lots of painful gas without constipation, you may have a food intolerance. Consult your doctor.

# How Can I Learn Some Techniques to Prepare Delicious Fruits and Vegetables?

Contained in the pages of this book are many easy recipes to help you prepare nutritious, delicious fruit and vegetable dishes. There are several key recipes that teach a cooking or preparation technique that can be applied to a variety of different ingredients. In other words, you can learn a few techniques that enable you to make hundreds of different healthy dishes.

---

## *Summary*

It is vitally important to your health to eat at least five to nine servings of fruits and vegetables a day. In order to do this here are some points to consider:

1. Eat fruits and vegetables throughout the day starting with breakfast.
2. Eat a variety of colorful fruits and vegetables. The more vibrant the colors the better. Try to include as many of the super phytonutrient containing fruits and veggies listed above in your daily diet.
3. Substitute fruits and vegetables for empty calories like French fries, processed snack foods, white breads, white pastas, white rice, and sodas.
4. Think out of the box when it comes to snacking in order to get more fruits and vegetables in your diet. Consider mini meals.
5. Make a habit of eating soup or salad for lunch.
6. Learn to prepare your own vegetables quickly and efficiently using recipes in this book.
7. Take a daily multivitamin.

---

# CHAPTER 11

# The Power of Protein

## *How to Feel Satisfied but Not Stuffed*

Protein is essential to every cell in the body. Next to water, the body contains more protein than any other substance. It's the body's structural building material as well as the body's all-important chemical messenger that spells out our DNA and our hormones and enzymes.

Proteins are made of just twenty different amino acid building blocks. These amino acids combine to form over ten thousand different proteins, each with a specific purpose. Luckily, we don't have to find all those different proteins in the foods we eat. The body has an amazing ability to make the proteins we need from the amino acid building blocks in our food and to recycle proteins we don't need by breaking them down into amino acids we can use.

The amino acids can be divided into two different types: essential and nonessential. Nonessential amino acids can be made by the body and don't have to be found in the diet pre-formed. Essential amino acids, however, cannot be made by the body and must come from the foods we eat. Almost all foods contain some protein, but all foods do not contain the nine essential amino acids in the proportions that we need. Foods that are deficient in the essential amino acids are considered to be *incomplete or low quality proteins*. Foods that have significant amounts of the nine essential amino acids are considered to be *complete or high quality proteins*.

Animal sources of protein, including dairy products, are complete proteins. Plant sources, with the exception of the soybean, are incomplete, but can become a complete protein when combined with a complementary protein source, like grains. Some examples of complementary proteins are lentils and rice, peanut butter and bread, and beans and tortillas.

Because protein is in most of the foods we eat, protein deficiency in this country is rare. Adults need to eat about half a gram of protein for every pound of lean body weight daily. If you're sedentary, like most Americans, that translates to about fifty grams of protein a day for the adult female and about sixty-five grams a day for the adult male. Growing children, pregnant and lactating women, and those who are participating in rigorous muscle-building physical activity need somewhat more than half a gram per pound per day. The body cannot store protein, so eating more protein than you need serves no purpose other than adding calories to your diet. Most of us don't need extra calories.

Consider that six ounces of lean chicken, beef or fish has between thirty-five and fifty grams of high quality protein (70 percent to 100 percent of the average woman's RDA), and a single cup of skim milk has 8.4 grams (17 percent of the average woman's RDA. Three cups contain one half of a woman's daily protein needs.). Two cups of skim milk contain about 75 percent of a four-year-old's protein needs. So don't worry if your child doesn't eat meat. Even vegetarians can easily get enough protein from their diet. Just two glasses of milk, a peanut butter sandwich, a cup of yogurt, plus a large serving of rice and beans contains over fifty grams of protein. Short of starvation or bizarre fad diets, it's difficult to be protein deficient in America.

However, the body cannot store the amino acid building blocks for later use. The body uses the protein we eat to build muscle, make enzymes, hormones, and other proteins, or uses them as fuel for energy. You must eat enough quality protein throughout the day or your body will start breaking down muscle to make the proteins it needs. This is quite counter productive if you want to lose weight, because muscle increases your metabolism and the amount of calories your burn.

*You must eat enough quality protein throughout the day or your body will start breaking down muscle to make the proteins it needs. This is quite counter productive if you want to lose weight, because muscle increases your metabolism and the amount of calories your burn.*

It's important to eat high quality protein or combine lower quality proteins to make complete protein at each meal and at most snacks. Not only does this ensure that you get enough amino acid building blocks to make the proteins you need without breaking down muscle, but it makes each meal and snack more satisfying. Protein also slows digestion of carbohydrates and thereby blunts the glycemic response to those carbohydrates. A meal that combines protein and carbohydrates causes a more gradual influx of glucose into the blood stream and less of a rise in insulin than a carbohydrate meal. This means that you take longer to get hungry again, even if you consume fewer calories.

*It's important to eat high quality protein or combine lower quality proteins to make complete protein at each meal and at most snacks.*

While it's easy to get enough protein, little is known about the effects of too much protein and how much is too much. High-protein, low-carbohydrate diets have gained recent popularity. It's true that high-protein diets can help you lose weight initially, but most people gain back the weight they lost when they start to eat carbohydrates again.

Recent studies show that high protein diets that cause ketosis, an abnormal biochemical state, can actually leave your fat cells more likely to accumulate stored fat. The long-term effects of high-protein diets are not well studied. Over time, excessive protein intake can cause loss of calcium from bone, which can result in brittle bones. A high-protein diet is also stressful to the kidneys and liver, espe-

> *It's true that high-protein diets can help you lose weight initially, but most people gain back the weight they lost when they start to eat carbohydrates again.*

cially if they're diseased. We don't know how much excess protein you would have to consume to damage normal kidneys and liver. However, because the body doesn't store protein per se, eating protein in excess of what's needed to make the body's proteins is just overeating. A diet moderate in protein is wise.

Rather than worrying about precisely *how much* protein to eat, it's more worthwhile to consider the *source* of protein in your diet. Protein seldom comes in a package by itself, so looking at the complete protein package is important. High-quality protein comes from animal sources packaged with varying amounts of saturated fats. Plant proteins are not usually complete proteins, but come packaged with carbohydrates, vitamins, phytonutrients and healthy fats.

## Should I Become a Vegetarian?

Whether or not to eat meat is a personal decision. It's more of a philosophical issue than a nutritional one. There's no *nutritional* reason to give up meat entirely, but plenty of nutritional reasons to *limit* your intake of animal foods and to choose them wisely.

Eating vegetable sources of protein the majority of the time will make it easier for you to lose excess weight or maintain a healthy weight, avoid environmental toxins, limit excess saturated fat, and ensure that you get plenty of fiber, antioxidants, and folate.

Nuts and nut butters are a complete, high quality protein and a good source of fiber, vitamins, iron, magnesium, and healthy fats. While nuts do have a lot of calories and fat, replacing meat or other carbohydrates in your diet with nuts can actually promote weight loss. Eating one to two ounces a day in place of animal protein or other carbohydrates is a great way to improve your health.

Bean and grain combinations are staples and comfort foods in cultures around the world for good reason. Beans are rich in protein, energy, iron, zinc, fiber, and antioxidants. Beans do need to be eaten with grains or dairy products to be a complete, high quality protein; however, beans count as both a vegetable and a protein source, making it easier to get all of your nutritional needs from fewer calories.

Soybeans and soy products, like soy milk and tofu, are complete proteins. Some soy products are even supplemented with calcium to increase their nutritional value.

There is no proof that one source of protein, animal or vegetable, is better for you than another. Ideally, you would base your diet on plant proteins with two to three daily servings of low-fat dairy products, and small amounts of animal proteins, like fish, eggs, and lean meats, to add variety, flavor, and extra iron and zinc.

Be careful choosing your animal protein. They are high quality, but come packaged with saturated fat and possible contaminants, like mercury in fish and hormones in milk. If you choose to eat meat, the issue of saturated fat can be tempered by eating small amounts of lean meat. A serving is generally the size and thickness of a deck of playing cards. Selecting lean cuts of meat and removing the skin and visible fat from meat and poultry before cooking reduces the amount of saturated fat in the package. Eating meat that has been fed a natural diet, such as grass-fed beef, also decreases the amount of saturated fat you eat because those animals tend to be leaner.

*A serving is generally the size and thickness of a deck of playing cards.*

Eating fish two to three times a week provides a high-quality protein source *and* omega-3 fatty acids; however, some fish are heavily contaminated with mercury from the environment.

- Large predatory fish like shark, tilefish, swordfish, and king mackerel tend to be the most contaminated (mercury concentration greater than .7 parts per million) and should be eaten rarely or avoided entirely.
- Fresh tuna, canned albacore tuna, red snapper, orange roughy, marlin, grouper, croaker, bluefish, halibut, saltwater bass, and sea trout have intermediate mercury levels (.2 to .7 ppm) and should be eaten in moderation, no more than once or twice a month.
- Salmon, cod, sardines, perch, haddock, whitefish, and tilapia, canned chunk light tuna, freshwater trout, and flounder are good choices. They usually have the lowest mercury levels and are generally safe to eat two to three times a week.

A recent study in the *New England Journal of Medicine* showed that men with high levels of mercury had about twice the incidence of heart attacks as those with lower levels. In other words, when it comes to heart attack prevention, highly contaminated fish are not a worthwhile source of omega-3s. The risks may outweigh the benefits. Pregnant women and children should be particularly cautious about eating contaminated fish. Mercury can damage the developing brains of children and fetuses.

*If we eat lots of animal products, we're placing ourselves at the top of the food chain, concentrating environmental toxins in our bodies. Eating a varied plant-based diet makes the accumulation of environmental contaminants and toxins in our bodies less likely.*

Eating at the top of the food chain is risky business. Toxins build up in the bodies of the animals at the top of the food chain because they eat many smaller less contaminated animals, but once their toxins are deposited in the fatty tissues of the body they're not easily eliminated. If we eat lots of animal products, we're placing ourselves at the top of the food chain, concentrating environmental toxins in our bodies. Eating a varied plant-based diet makes the accumulation of environmental contaminants and toxins in our bodies less likely.

## When I Eat Meat or Dairy Products, Does It Matter How the Animal Was Raised?

Absolutely. Most animals raised for meat or dairy products are raised inhumanely. They are not allowed to roam free and eat their healthy natural diet, be it grass or insects or vegetables. They're often raised in overcrowded warehouses where they are caged or tethered most of their lives in front of a feed trough full of grain, soy meal, bakery waste, chicken manure, pesticide-laced fruits and vegetables, and other things they would not naturally eat. Aside from the obvious cruelty of treating animals this way, these unnatural practices have undesirable effects on the animals' meat as well as the milk or eggs they produce.

*Cows and chickens allowed to roam free and eat natural foods have meat with healthier nutritional profiles.*

Cows and chickens allowed to roam free and eat natural foods have meat with healthier nutritional profiles. They contain less saturated fat and more omega-3 fatty acids than caged animals fed the scrap and supplement diet so commonly used these days. Grass-fed beef contains less saturated fat as well as less arachidonic acid, a fatty acid contained in red meat and egg yolks that's harmful when eaten in excess. Chickens fed flaxseed meal high in omega-3 fatty acids produce eggs high in omega-3 fatty acids. Chickens fed monotonous diets of grain rather than a natural variety of grasses, insects, and seeds produce less flavorful, vitamin-depleted eggs with less healthy fat profiles.

"You are what you eat" applies to animals as well as humans. The quality of fish is also affected by their diet. Farm-raised fish that are fed soy and corn rather than their natural aquatic diet often have less favorable fat profiles. Farm-raised Atlantic salmon has significantly more harmful arachidonic acid than wild salmon. Look for Coho Salmon (farmed or wild), canned salmon, or wild Atlantic salmon for the best omega-3 to arachidonic acid ratios. Atlantic cod, Atlantic and Pacific halibut, and farmed catfish have significantly less omega-3s than their counterparts— Pacific cod, Greenland halibut, and wild catfish.

Feeding cows diets primarily of grains with little of the green vegetation that they would normally eat makes them fat. This is good if you're a farmer trying to get as much meat as possible from your investment, but it's not good for the planet or the person who ends up eating the meat. The meat of grain-fed beef has more saturated fat than the meat of grass-fed beef. It takes much more natural resources to feed a cow grain than grass. It wastes even more natural resources for humans to eat grain-fed cattle instead of eating the grain and vegetables themselves. Large parts of the world have been devoted to feeding and pasturing livestock. Only a fraction of this land would be necessary to feed the world a vegetarian diet. In addition, livestock wastes are major contributors to groundwater pollution as well as the greenhouse effect.

Cows are often injected with growth hormones that increase milk production. These hormones can be excreted into their milk. Since bovine growth hormones have only been used since 1994, long-term effects on humans who drink the growth hormone-containing milk are not yet known, but there may be an association between bovine growth hormone and human cancer.

Animals including farmed fish, cattle, swine, and poultry raised under unnatural conditions are treated frequently with antibiotics to protect them from bacterial diseases that are common in overcrowded, squalid living conditions. These antibiotics treat the same bacteria that make humans sick. Overtreatment with antibiotics leads to the development of stronger bacteria that are no longer killed by the overused antibiotics. When these bacteria infect us, our antibiotics are useless against them. Bacterial resistance to antibiotics has become a worldwide problem.

## Savvy Eating Info: What Is Arachidonic Acid?

Arachidonic acid (AA) is a fatty acid found in animal flesh, egg yolks, and human milk. It's essential to the body in small amounts. Eating large amounts of AA can cause susceptible people to have trouble with inflammatory diseases like arthritis, heart disease, allergies, and asthma. While AA is good for infants' development (it is added to infant formula!), as you get older, you become more sensitive to AA and need to cut down on foods with high AA content.

In general, this can be done by eating a more plant-based diet, eating only lean meats, eating animals that were raised on natural diets, avoiding Atlantic *farm-raised* salmon (yes salmon!), and limiting the number of egg yolks you eat. It's a good idea to make your omelets whiter as you grow older. Feed kids whole eggs. Transition to two egg whites for every egg yolk in the teen years and use more egg whites as an adult.

*Why Avoid Salmon? I Thought It Was Supposed To Be Good for Me.*
Surprisingly, some fish contain more AA than any other food. However, when the amount of AA a fish contains is balanced with the amount it has of eicosapentaenoic acid or EPA (an omega-3 fatty acid found in fish), the body runs well. Unfortunately, some fish, like *farm-raised* Atlantic salmon, Chinook salmon, sea trout, whiting, pompano, non-Greenland halibut and eel have lots of AA without much EPA to balance it out. When the amount of AA is much greater than the amount of EPA you eat, you can become prone to inflammation.

*My Picks for Safe Fish (Low in Mercury) that Are High in*
*EPA and Low in AA*

- Anchovies, *wild* catfish, *Pacific* cod, fish sticks made from cod or perch (make sure there are no added trans fats), flounder, haddock, *Greenland* halibut, herring, perch, *canned* salmon, *Coho* salmon (farmed or wild), *Atlantic Wild* Salmon, *Atlantic* sardines, *canned* light or white tuna, *freshwater* trout, whitefish, *wild* shrimp, blue crab, and Alaskan king crab are generally safe from mercury contamination and have more EPA than AA.

(Based on the USDA nutrient database 17 and the USFDA 2004 tables of Mercury Levels in Commercial Fish and Shellfish)

> ### Savvy Eating Info: Vegan Diets
>
> Vegan diets (no meat, eggs, dairy, or animal products of any kind) are undertaken for philosophical reasons only, as they have no nutritional rationale. While vegan diets are good for the environment, they're unnatural for humans and can lead to deficiencies in vitamins D, B12, and B2, calcium, iron, and zinc, which then need to be taken as supplements.

Whenever possible, choose meat, fish, poultry, eggs, and dairy products that are raised without antibiotics or hormones, and on natural diets under humane conditions. This helps the animals themselves, our own health, and the planet as a whole. If humanely raised products are not available where you live, or simply too expensive, consider eating fewer animal products.

## Does It Matter How I Cook the Meat I Eat?

Probably. Carcinogenic compounds called heterocyclic amines are generated when meat is cooked at high temperatures as when grilling or frying meat to a well-done state. We don't know how much of these compounds it takes to have serious consequences, but it's probably a good idea to get out the crock-pot every now and then, and grill and pan fry less often. Don't eat blackened meat.

*If you like to eat red meat, you can trim all visible fat then marinate it in a combination of red wine and olive oil for twenty-four hours prior to cooking it. The red wine leaches out some of the saturated fat and arachidonic acid in the meat and replaces it with healthy fat from the olive oil.*

If you like to eat red meat, you can trim all visible fat then marinate it in a combination of red wine and olive oil for twenty-four hours prior to cooking it. The red wine leaches out some of the saturated fat and arachidonic acid in the meat and replaces it with healthy fat from the olive oil. This method also gives the meat a wonderful taste and texture. Try grass-fed beef and bison. They're much better for you and taste great. Bison is particularly tasty and has a healthier fat profile. There are no growth hormones in bison, and they don't get mad cow disease.

# What about Eggs?

Eggs are a neat little package of high-quality protein, iron, vitamin D, and healthy nutrients like choline and caritenoids, but they also contain saturated fat, arachidonic acid, and cholesterol. In general, it's considered safe to eat an egg a day (including the eggs you eat in baked goods), but for healthy active individuals, somewhat more is probably OK. The saturated fat and arachdonic acid in the egg is contained in the yolk. If you want to eat more than an egg a day, consider substituting two egg whites for each whole egg for some or all of the eggs in baked goods, omelets, and other dishes.

# Do I Need To Drink Milk?

Milk can be a part of a healthy diet as long as you drink skim milk. Whole milk should only be consumed by toddlers between the ages of twelve months and two years who still need the extra fat for brain development. Infants below twelve months should not eat dairy products at all, and children over the age of two should drink skim milk like the rest of the family.

The designations ½ percent, 1 percent and 2 percent refer to the percentage of milk fat by weight. Consider that whole milk (3 percent to 4 percent fat by weight) has 150 calories per cup, and 50 percent of those calories are from fat; 2 percent milk has 120 calories per cup, and 35 percent of its calories come from fat.. Skim milk has about ninety calories per cup and is fat free. It's an excellent source of calcium and high-quality protein, and in this country, it's fortified with vitamin D.

Vitamin D is as important as calcium when it comes to bone strengthening. Vitamin D is made naturally when our skin is exposed to at least fifteen minutes of sunlight a few times a week. Many people with dark skin or who live in northern climates (latitudes north of Philadelphia) don't get enough sunlight to make sufficient amounts of vitamin D, which can lead to osteoporosis or rickets without supplementation.

Other dairy products like yogurt and cheese are also good protein and calcium sources, but often come packaged with saturated fat or extra sugar. Sweetened yogurts are an unusually high source of empty calories from sugar. Cheeses have a lot of saturated fat. Dairy products other than milk are not necessarily supplemented with vitamin D. Check the label.

Healthy adults can benefit from consuming about two to three servings of skim milk or low-fat dairy products a day. Except during adolescence, lactation, and pregnancy when three or more servings are recommended, it's probably safest to limit your dairy intake to three servings a day. Those who drink too much milk are often constipated. High consumption of milk has, in a few studies, been linked with ovarian and prostate cancer. However, too little calcium is dangerous too. Low calcium intake has been linked with osteoporosis, obesity, and high blood pressure. Moderation is key. While you can get your calcium from a number of other sources, like supplements, milk substitutes, or other foods, calcium from dairy products seems to help control weight better than calcium from other sources.

# What If I Don't Eat Dairy Products?

For those who don't tolerate dairy products either because of allergy, lactose intolerance, or because they just don't like the taste, there are plenty of other ways to ensure healthy bones. Unless you consume at least two or three servings of dairy products or fortified milk substitutes daily, you should take a multivitamin containing vitamin D and calcium. Most multivitamins contain about one-third of your RDA, so you will have to get the rest of your calcium from other foods like fortified tofu, soy milk, cereals, beans, or green vegetables, or from calcium supplements. No matter how much calcium you get in your diet, you won't build stronger bones unless you also get enough vitamin D to help form strong bones, enough vitamin K (found in green leafy vegetables) to stabilize bone and prevent bone loss, and get regular vigorous weight-bearing exercise.

---

### Savvy Eating Tips: Help for the Lactose Intolerant

If you're one of the many people who get gas, bloating, cramps, or diarrhea when you drink milk, you may be able to eat small portions of dairy products without symptoms. Many who can't digest lactose can eat small servings of yogurt or hard cheese without problems. However, those who get symptoms from even small amounts of dairy can often tolerate dairy food if they take a "lactase" enzyme supplement with each serving of dairy food. There are many brands available at drug stores and health food stores. Some brands also contain other proteases (digestive enzymes) and beneficial probiotic organisms that may further aid digestion.

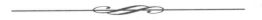

## *Summary*

Protein is abundant in our food supply. It's vitally important to our bodies and gives us long-lasting satiety. It's a good idea to eat a source of high-quality protein at every meal and snack if possible. We just need to choose our protein sources wisely.

1. Choose plant sources of protein like nuts, soy products, and beans in place of animal products often.
2. When you do eat red meat or pork, choose lean cuts and trim visible fat. Remove the skin from poultry before cooking and eat white meat.
3. Whenever possible, choose animal products that have been raised humanely on natural diets without the use of hormones or antibiotics.
4. Choose skim milk and non-fat yogurt over other dairy products and limit intake to three servings a day (unless you're a teenager, or pregnant or lactating).
5. Eat non-predatory fish two to three times a week.
6. Eat a serving of protein with every meal and most snacks.

# CHAPTER 12

# A Sense of Portion

## *Knowing When Enough Is Enough*

Developing a sense of portion size is one of the most important concepts in healthy eating. Not only does portion size play a vital role in keeping your body weight stable and healthy, but it also enables you to eat enough of the nutrients your body needs, while limiting the amount of empty calories and harmful substances you eat.

Most Americans are used to large portions. This is due, in part, to the fact that about one-third of us eat out daily. Restaurant servings, especially in fast-food restaurants are increasingly oversized. The restaurant items that tend to be most oversized are salty fried foods, white breads, and sweet drinks. These are all foods that are best avoided in the first place, not foods that are necessary parts of our diet. Fruits, vegetables, and whole grains, however, are dramatically under-represented in restaurant foods as well as in our own homes.

When I ask patients how many servings of fruits and vegetables they eat each day, they often answer five a day. However, when I ask which ones they ate over the past twenty-four hours, it goes something like this: "I had a glass of orange juice, jelly on my sandwich, and fruit yogurt. I ate a burger with lettuce, tomato, and pickle, and French fries." By my count, that's a little under two servings of fruits and vegetables. Let me explain why.

Orange juice is a legitimate vitamin, mineral, and phytonutrient-containing serving of fruit. However, it lacks the fiber that would be contained in an actual orange. Juices have a high glycemic index and are not as satisfying as the fruits from which they came. Juices should be limited to one six- to eight-ounce serving a day for the average adult (and four to six ounces a day for children) because the calories add up quickly without filling you up. Eating the whole fruit is better.

The amount of fruit in jelly, fruit yogurt, or even fruit leathers, like fruit roll-ups and so forth, or fruited muffins is negligible. A fruit yogurt generally has less than one to two tablespoons of fruit and a lot of added sugar. That's about one-eighth of a serving.

The burger toppings aren't much help either. The lettuce leaf on the burger is probably less than one-eighth of a serving of leafy greens. (A standard one-cup serving of leafy greens should cover a dinner plate, not just your burger.) The anemic looking slice of tomato is about another one-eighth of a serving, and the pickle probably is not worth mentioning.

French fries are in a category unto themselves. Most nutrition experts would not recommend counting fries as a vegetable at all. For one thing, it takes very little potato to make a bag of fries. Even a six-ounce super-size fries serving contains about half of a large potato without its vitamin-, mineral-, and fiber-containing skin. Just to make matters worse, most fries are fried in partially hydrogenated oils. Also, potatoes are fairly unique in the vegetable world in that they have a very high glycemic index. Fries are not a food I would count toward your daily fruit and vegetable intake. Unfortunately, fried potatoes are the most popular vegetable in the U.S.

Clearly the patient whose diet I described above was not getting sufficient amounts of fruits and vegetables, but she thought she was doing OK. She assumed that she was getting five servings of fruits and vegetables when she was actually just getting five tastes of fruits and vegetables.

Many of us make portion errors in the opposite direction. It's easy to do with today's super-sizing. We often get many more servings of refined carbohydrates than we think. Most people think of a bagel or the two slices of bread that enclose our sandwich as being one serving; however, they are two servings. A large, white sub roll can be four servings of nutritionally empty calories. A thirty-two-ounce soda is also four servings of empty carbohydrate calories.

Some feel that a restaurant steak would constitute a serving; however, steaks are often two, three, or even four three-ounce servings. Serving size for protein is not a one-size-fits-all situation. Your protein requirements depend on your size (lean body mass), your level of activity, and whether or not you're growing.

For example, a sedentary 250-pound man will need less protein than a 145-pound active teenager. An overweight 150-pound person will require less protein than a fit 135-pound active person will. A good rule of thumb is that you should eat a source of complete protein (like milk, meat, eggs, cheese, nuts, seeds, soy products, or a plant protein combination like rice and beans) at every meal and at most snacks.

As mentioned above, your protein portion size depends on your size, activity level, and whether you are growing. You can use what I call the "rule of hand" to determine how much protein you need to eat at each meal.

It's also helpful to have an idea of relative portion size. When you

---

### Savvy Eating Tips: The Rule of Hand for Protein

- In general, a portion of *lean beef, pork, or poultry* should be about the size and thickness of the palm of your hand (not including the fingers and thumb). You can eat lean meats up to twice a day, but less is desirable.
- A portion of *fish* should be the size and thickness of your whole hand. Enjoy fish two to three times a week.
- A portion of *eggs* will fit into the palm of your cupped hand (that's about two eggs or one egg plus two egg whites for the average adult). Eat up to seven whole eggs a week.
- A serving of *milk* is eight ounces. A serving of cheese is a one-inch cube. Get two to three servings a day for the average adult.
- A serving of *nuts* covers half of the surface of your palm. A serving of peanut butter is the size of a golf ball. These are healthy but calorie dense foods. Limit yourself to two servings a day, most days.
- Vegetarians will need to eat a large serving of complete protein at every meal and most snacks. Plant sources of protein such as beans with grains and tofu double as vegetables and grains, so you can usually eat as much of them as you care to eat.

If you're still growing or very active, your portion size will be larger than those listed above. If you're sedentary, your portion size will be somewhat smaller. At each meal, start with a serving of protein as described above. Remember, you don't have to clean your plate.

---

look at your dinner plate, vegetables and fruits should cover at least half of it. Your portion of animal protein should follow the "rule of hand," and your portion of whole grains and/or starches should be about the same size as your protein.

For most Americans, following these guidelines will call for much larger portions of vegetables and much smaller portions of grains and starches. For example, if you consider the American staple, the hamburger and fries, under these guidelines you would eat a hamburger patty the size of your palm (a smaller one if you want cheese on it) and a bun that is no bigger than the hamburger patty. For most of us that's half of a large bun or one small bun. That leaves no room

*It's also helpful to have an idea of relative portion size. When you look at your dinner plate, vegetables and fruits should cover at least half of it. Your portion of animal protein should follow the "rule of hand," and your portion of whole grains and/or starches should be about the same size as your protein.*

for French fries! The rest of your plate should be filled with baked beans, roasted vegetables, salad, or other fruits and vegetables.

*Savvy Eating does not mean depriving yourself of the foods that you love, it means you need to eat smaller portions of foods that are not good for you and larger portions of foods that make you healthy.*

If you can't do without the fries, skip the bun and opt for fries fried in healthy oils and limit yourself to a portion the same size as your palm. Savvy Eating does not mean depriving yourself of the foods that you love, it means you need to eat smaller portions of foods that are not good for you and larger portions of foods that make you healthy. Eat foods that contain grains, starches, sweets, and saturated fats in moderation, while filling up on satisfying foods like luscious salads with tasty dressings, nuts, fruits, and lean proteins.

In order to eat well, it's important to have a good grasp of what a serving of food should look like. For most of us that takes a brief period of actually measuring out a serving of our most commonly eaten foods and seeing what that serving looks like on the dish or in the container that we will usually see them. Measure out one-half cup of grapes and see what they look like in your hand. Measure out one-half cup of cooked carrots and put them on your plate next to your chicken. A standard ice cream scoop is about one-quarter cup when filled level to the rim, not heaping. (A heaping scoop of ice cream is closer to one-half cup.)

---

### Savvy Eating Tips: The Three Bears Had the Right Idea

Papa Bear had a great big bowl, Mama Bear had a medium-sized bowl, and Baby Bear had a wee little bowl.

Studies show that the size of our bowls, plates, and cups plays a roll in determining how large a serving we take. More importantly, the amount of food on our plates greatly influences how much we eat.

In a study, people were served small or large portions of food and allowed to eat as much as they wanted. Those who were served a small portion, tended to eat less than those who were served a larger portion. Surprisingly, satisfaction ratings were similar in both the large portion and the small portion groups.

If you're trying to lose weight, use slightly smaller plates. Serve kids on kid-sized plates. Serve tea, soda, and juice in small cups. Use large cups for water. Use big soup bowls and salad plates, and small plates for dessert.

As you get older, you may want to down-size your every day plates and bowls as your metabolism downsizes. Using oversized plates can actually lead to overeating!

Use the scoop to serve grains and veggies to give yourself a quick gage of how big your servings are.

When you prepare a pasta dish with vegetables in it, take out the vegetables just once and see if your serving of pasta contains a serving of vegetables. Are you getting a serving of vegetables or just a taste of them? Are you getting more servings of carbohydrates than you thought? Is your protein portion proportional to your body size and activity level?

Try to measure all of the foods you routinely eat during the two weeks that you keep your food journal. (Try to avoid measuring at the table. Your meal will be more relaxed and pleasurable if you do it while you are preparing the meal if possible.) Measuring the amount of food you eat is an inconvenience, but it's temporary and very helpful. Measuring becomes unnecessary once you've gotten an eye for portion size, but you may want to measure occasionally as you add new foods to your diet. Use the following chart to check the serving size of various foods. Once you become familiar with what a serving size is, you can determine whether you're getting enough healthy foods or too many nutritionally empty foods.

### General Chart of Serving Sizes for Adults

| Type of food | | Serving size |
| --- | --- | --- |
| Fruits (include at least 2–3 daily) | Melons, and other large watery fruits | 1 cup |
| | Apples, pears, oranges, peaches, and other medium-sized fruits | 1 medium-sized whole fruit |
| | Grapes and berries | ½ cup |
| | Dried fruits | ¼ cup |
| | Fruit and vegetable juices | ¾ cup (6 ounces) |
| Vegetables (include at least 3–6 daily) | Leafy green, raw | 1 cup |
| | Other raw vegetables | ½ cup |
| | Cooked, including legumes | ½ cup |
| Dairy (include 2–3 daily) | Milk | 8 ounces |
| | Cheese | 1 ounce (about a 1-inch cube for most cheeses or the size of a 9-volt battery) |
| | Yogurt | 8 ounces (1 cup) |
| Meats (include up to 1 or 2 a day) | Red meat, pork, poultry, fish (Remember bacon is not a meat, it's a fat) | A portion of meat or poultry is the size and thickness of the palm of your hand, *excluding* the fingers (3 to 4 ounces for most adults). |

*(continued)*

| Type of food | | Serving size |
|---|---|---|
| | | Fish portions are a little less than the size of your whole hand, *including* fingers (4 to 6 ounces) |
| | Eggs | 2 whole or 1 whole and 2 egg whites |
| Grains | Rice, oats, and other whole grains, cooked | ¾ cup cooked oatmeal (½-cup uncooked oats) or ½-cup cooked rice (¼-cup uncooked rice, barley, or other grains) |
| | Breads | ½ small bagel, 1 slice of bread, 1 small muffin, ⅓ bakery muffin, ½ pastry, ¼ (6″) sub roll, ½ hamburger or hotdog roll, ½ pita, 1 small tortilla, ¼₄ cake or 1 small cupcake (no frosting), 1 (4″) pancake (the same size as a DVD) |
| | Pasta, cooked | ½ cup (one heaping ice cream scoop) |
| | Dry cereals | ½ to 1 cup (amount that contains 15 to 25 grams of carbohydrate; read the label.) |
| Processed foods | | See package information |

# How Much Fat Do I Need?

Getting the right amount of fat in your diet is a little more ambiguous. Other than actively avoiding trans fats and limiting saturated fats as much as possible by choosing low-fat dairy products and lean meats, there are no hard and fast rules on fat portions. By and large, fats are not foods that we consume on their own. They are usually consumed as a part of another food, either because they're a natural part of that food, like the oils contained in fish or oats, or it's added to a food to increase its palatability, like dressing on a salad.

If you eat lean meats and low-fat dairy products, you can enjoy the fats that occur naturally in fruits, vegetables, and grains and add moderate amounts of healthy fats to your foods without worry. The recipes in this book offer delicious vegetables, salads, breads, entrees, and even desserts with a reasonable amount of healthy fats. The amount of fat in fried foods, full-fat dairy products, and most commercial cakes, cookies, and many home-baked goods is excessive and should be limited or avoided entirely.

Adding two or three tablespoons of dressing made with olive or canola oil to your salad is reasonable. Drenching your salad in ½-cup of bleu cheese dressing is not. Cooking your veggies in a few teaspoons of olive oil enhances their flavor. Dipping your pizza crust in garlic butter is too much.

# The Cardinal Rule: Do Not Overeat

Eating moderate amounts of healthy fats and unrefined grains while eating a source of protein at each meal and most snacks, and eating plenty of fruits and vegetables will undoubtedly make your diet healthy. However, you won't achieve optimum health unless you obey the most important rule: Do not overeat! No chart or calculation, no matter how meticulous, can tell you know precisely how much you need to eat. They can only provide guidelines. You must cultivate awareness of your own satisfaction.

*You won't achieve optimum health unless you obey the most important rule: Do not overeat! No chart or calculation, no matter how meticulous, can tell you precisely how much you need to eat. They can only provide guidelines. You must cultivate awareness of your own satisfaction.*

For some this comes quite naturally, and for others, it takes some practice. Those who maintain appropriate weight have usually mastered the ability to stop eating when satisfied. Those who are overweight may have one of three problems or a combination of the three:

1. They eat *too many calorie-dense foods*, like sweets, fried foods, refined snack foods, nuts, fatty meats and cheese.
2. They eat *too many low nutrient density foods* like sweet drinks, cookies, white breads, and pretzels that lack satisfying healthy fats, fiber, and protein.
3. They *eat past the point of feeling satisfied*.

Eating a diet high in fruits, vegetables, whole grains, lean proteins, and healthy fats will help you stay satisfied between meals and snacks, but it's up to you to stop eating when you are satisfied, *before* you are full.

Awareness of satiety can take time to develop. When in doubt, stop eating as soon as you no longer feel hungry and do something else. Wait at least thirty minutes before deciding if you're still hungry. You can always have a healthy snack later if you feel hungry before the next meal. If

your work from your desk, take a deep breath or give thanks before you begin to eat, and eat your snack as peacefully and mindfully as possible. When you're done, clear all snack remnants from your desk and resume your work. You'll feel much more satisfied having eaten this way than if you had taken bites of an apple or spoonfuls of yogurt between tasks. Your desk will be much neater too. If you're concerned about the time you'll lose from work while taking a break to eat, consider that it rarely takes more than two minutes to eat a snack. You'll easily make up for the lost time through the increased productivity that follows eating mindfully.

# Thinking Outside the Box: What to Eat for Snacks

Nutritious snacks are as important as nutritious meals. Unfortunately, Americans rarely think beyond the snack options that are available in the vending machine or the snack food aisle of the grocery store. While prepackaged foods are convenient, they're not usually healthy choices. One major exception is prepackaged nuts, which are satisfying and healthy.

*Nutritious snacks are as important as nutritious meals.*

Convenience, nutrition, and satisfaction are not too much to demand of your snack food. Because healthy foods are not always available at work, school, or on the road, healthy snacking does take some forethought. Plan your snacks. Buy the healthy snack foods of your choice in bulk and keep them in your office and home.

Fresh fruit and vegetables are the ideal snack food, especially if you only need your snack to tide you over an hour or two until your next meal. Keep a bowl of fresh fruit in your office and at home. If fruit is in plain sight, you are more likely to snack on it. Prepare several days' worth of vegetable sticks at one time for yourself and the whole family and put them in plastic bags in the refrigerator. If refrigeration is not available at work or at school, an insulated lunchbox and an ice pack will keep perishables cold.

*Keep a bowl of fresh fruit in your office and at home. If fruit is in plain sight, you are more likely to snack on it.*

If the thought of fresh fruit and veggies as your only snack options give you the sudden urge to drive to a convenience store for chips, then you may need to make other healthy snack choices. Nuts are a perfect snack food especially if it will be a long time until your next meal. They contain fiber, protein, and healthy fats that keep you satisfied for a long time. They're a good replacement for unhealthy, salty, and crunchy snacks like chips. Trail mix is another good option. Just make sure that the one you choose is not made with partially hydrogenated oils.

Be mindful of portion size with high calorie foods like nuts and trail mix. You might want to put snack-sized portions in baggies, so you know when to quit. Popcorn can be a good snack if it's air popped or popped in a healthy oil, but microwave popcorns usually contain trans fats and should be avoided. Chips, pretzels, graham crackers, and cereal bars often contain refined grains, sugar, trans fats or just empty calories. If you can't do without them, opt for brands that are trans fat-free and list whole grains as the first ingredient. Homemade toasted whole-wheat pita chips dipped in peanut butter or bean dip, whole-grain cereal snack mix with nuts, and granola (in small portions) are other healthy snacks that can be made to suit your taste.

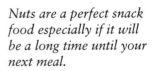

*Nuts are a perfect snack food especially if it will be a long time until your next meal.*

Non-fat yogurt or fruit smoothies are satisfying for those who like smooth and creamy snacks. Homemade smoothies that are made with large portions of fruit, fat-free yogurt, and a small amount of sweetener are best. Commercial smoothies are often too sweet and come in huge sizes. Opt for low- or non-fat and low-sugar varieties. If you sweeten plain yogurt with a little honey, you'll end up eating less sugar than you would if you ate a sweetened variety. Honey also has a lower glycemic index than sugar.

## Mini-Meals Improve Snack Quality

Another great option is to eat mini-meals. If you have four or five smaller meals in a day, you're less likely to overeat because you're too hungry, and you're more likely to eat nutritious foods like fruits and vegetables. Eating mini-meals might be right for you if you find yourself overeating when you snack. Plan to eat cereal, milk, and fruit in the morning, a salad or sandwich at eleven, a hearty soup at two or three, and then sit down with the family for fish and veggies in the evening. It doesn't take any longer to heat up a bowl of soup than it does to microwave popcorn for an afternoon snack. Choosing healthy snacks will help you keep your blood sugar steady and make you feel more energetic throughout the day.

## Keep Portions in Mind

How much you eat when you snack is also a major concern. It would be difficult to eat too much if you're snacking on orange slices or celery sticks, but eating can get out of hand with tasty nuts, trail mix, or a large fruit smoothie. Your snack only needs to supply enough energy to satisfy your hunger until you have your next meal.

If you tend to snack out of control when conventional snack foods are available, make sure they're not available on a regular basis. Don't buy them! Eat them as occasional treats, but don't keep them in the house. Three types of snacks are the usual culprits that tend to lead to overeating: sweets, salty foods, and foods with a variety of different tastes and shapes, such as snack mixes with cereal, pretzels, nuts, and crackers. If you're susceptible to overindulgence in these types of food, avoid them as snacks, or place a reasonable serving in an individual container and resolve to eat only that amount. Don't depend on will power alone; keep unhealthy snacks out of your house and plan ahead to have healthy snacks or mini-meals.

## *Summary*

1. Eat snacks mindfully without distraction.
2. Plan ahead to make healthy snacks convenient. Make the quality of your snacks as good as the quality of your meals.
3. Consider mini-meals in place of traditional snacks.
4. Keep portion size in mind, especially with healthy but calorie-dense foods like nuts, granola, trail mix, and smoothies.

# CHAPTER 14

# What to Drink

Beverages other than skim milk and water are expensive and not a necessary part of a healthy diet. If you like coffee, tea, red wine, beer, or juices, they can be a part of a healthy diet in moderation.

## Why Do We Need Milk?

Skim milk (not 1 percent, 2 percent, or whole milk) is an excellent source of protein and calcium that is free of saturated fat. Children aged two to eight should get two eight-ounce cups a day. People over age eight should get three servings. Pregnant and lactating women should get more. While we could easily eat other sources of protein, milk contains a bioavailable source of calcium that is vital for modern people's health. If you don't drink milk, you need to eat an equivalent amount of calcium from another source. Fat-free yogurt, fortified soy products and supplements are the best alternatives. Other dairy products, like cheese, are good sources, too. You can replace up to one milk serving a day with fortified juices, but I would not recommend more than one serving of juice a day.

Many dieters and nutritionists alike have debated our need for milk because it seems unnatural for one species to depend on the milk of another species. Ancient man probably didn't need to drink milk, but modern man has evolved to need it. There are four major reasons:

1. Modern man generally gets less sunlight, therefore less vitamin D, than our ancestors. Modern man benefits form vitamin D fortified milk to develop and maintain strong bones.
2. We get less exercise than our ancestors. Exercise is key in developing and maintaining healthy bones. Those who don't get daily weight-bearing exercise need all the bone-strengthening help they can get from fortified milk.
3. In general, modern man is taller and heavier than ancient man. Our bones are longer and more vulnerable to breakage, so we need extra calcium to prevent broken bones from falls.

4. We live longer than both our ancient ancestors and our ancestors from just a few decades ago. There was no need to worry
about osteoporosis and hip fractures in your seventies if you
only lived to be thirty-five. We need milk to preserve our bone
strength because so many people are living well into their seventies, eighties, and nineties.

## Coffee and Tea

Tea made fresh (tea loses its antioxidant power after several hours) and
without sweeteners is a very healthy addition to your diet because it
contains many antioxidants. Coffee also contains
many antioxidants. However, it's wise to drink tea
and coffee in moderation because they contain
caffeine in addition to antioxidants. Coffee can
also be irritating to the stomach, especially for
those who have reflux. It's a good idea to limit
your caffeinated coffee to two cups a day and tea
to three cups. If you like to drink more, consider
drinking some natural or water processed decaf-
feinated beverages. Even natural decaffeinating
processes remove some of the antioxidants, however.

> *Tea made fresh (tea loses its antioxidant power after several hours) and without sweeteners is a very healthy addition to your diet because it contains many antioxidants.*

## Fruit Juices

Juices are only a part of a healthy diet if they're consumed in moderation. If you're not overweight, one six- to eight-ounce serving (four to
six ounces for children under age six) of unsweetened 100 percent juice
can be beneficial, especially if you don't like whole fruit. If you're overweight, it's best to skip the juice and opt for whole fruits. Liquid calories
are much less satisfying than solid foods and promote overeating. Don't
be duped into buying fruit-flavored drinks. Drinks containing less than
100 percent fruit juice aren't worth drinking. Choose 100 percent juice
or water instead.

## Tap Water—The Best Drink of All

Most of the eight or more cups of liquid you need each day should be water. You need to drink enough water to make your urine clear, not yellow.

Most people don't get enough. Unless your community water supply is unsafe, you're better off drinking tap water than bottled water. Most bottled waters are taken from municipal water supplies much like your own, but they've been sitting around in plastic bottles leaching chemicals as well as that "plastic" taste out of the bottle and into the water you drink. They're also expensive. If you're concerned about unwanted impurities in your water, consider buying a reverse osmosis water purification system for your household. It will remove toxic metals, organic materials and minerals (as well as fluoride, so inform your dentist). The systems are expensive, sometimes slow, and do waste water.

If you just want water that tastes good, invest in one of the many, less expensive, carbon filter systems available in the grocery or discount store. Just be sure to change the filter as often as recommended to avoid bacterial build up. These filters also remove fluoride.

## No Place for Sodas

Sodas whether decaf, sugary, or artificially sweetened have no place in a healthy diet. Even if the caffeine and empty calories have been removed, carbonated beverages deplete our bones of calcium and harm our tooth enamel. What's more, Americans tend to drink sodas in place of milk or other calcium-containing beverages, making osteoporosis much more likely. Fifty percent of American teens don't get enough calcium. Don't waste your money and calories on beverages that don't benefit your body, or even worse, do your body harm. Adults and children alike benefit from replacing sodas with skim milk or water.

## What About Alcohol?

Moderate alcohol consumption does have some health benefits. It can increase HDL and help protect you from heart disease and stroke. Red wine in particular contains potent antioxidants. If you already drink beer or wine, drinking no more than one glass of wine or one bottle of beer no more three to four times a week can be a healthy choice. If you drink hard liquor or more than three to four servings of beer or wine a week, the toxic effects of alcohol begin to overbalance the positive effects of these beverages. If you do not drink alcohol, no need to start.

It's especially important not to drink alcohol if you are pregnant or have a personal or family history of alcoholism. Having a daily serving of concord grapes or concord grape juice can have similar benefits.

### Savvy Eating Tips: The "Taste" of Water

*I don't like the "taste" of water even if it is filtered.* Pure water has no taste. If you get a bad taste when you drink an unflavored beverage, chances are that the taste is actually coming from your mouth rather than your water. Going for long periods of time without drinking, drinking sweetened drinks, eating a high GL diet, and poor oral hygiene can cause the bacteria in your mouth to multiply rapidly. Waste products of these bacteria leave a putrid taste in your mouth that is more apparent when you take a sip of water, bringing those waste products from the crevices between your teeth to your tongue. If you think you don't like the taste of purified water, brush your teeth and drink more often. Your water might taste much better.

## *Summary*

1. Adults should drink at least eight eight-ounce glasses of water daily.
2. Fresh tea and coffee, red wine, and even beer can be beneficial in limited quantities.
3. Avoid sweetened drinks and carbonated beverages, but a daily serving of 100 percent fruit juice is OK.
4. Drink two to three servings of skim milk or milk substitutes a day as discussed in chapter 11.

# CHAPTER 15

# Eating Out: Menu Management

Peole who eat out tend to eat more saturated fat, calories, and refined carbohydrates than do those who eat at home. They also eat fewer fruits and vegetables. The more you eat out, the more likely you are to be overweight. Up to one third of Americans eat out once a day, so eating out is a significant nutritional issue. Therefore, it's smart to have a plan before you open the menu.

> *The more you eat out, the more likely you are to be overweight.*

## Fast Food

If you're eating at a fast-food restaurant, having a plan is easy because they don't vary their menus much. They also make nutritional information readily available if you ask for it. If you can't avoid eating fast food often, then get to know the menus at the fast-food establishments that you go to most frequently. Most fast-food chains specialize in meat and cheese on a white bun, served with French fries or chips, and copious amounts of sweetened beverages.

Some offer healthier options like salads, but they're not as healthy as the ones you would make at home. You still have to read their labels to look for trans fats, saturated fat, and refined carbohydrates. The vegetables they serve are not usually as fresh or vibrantly colored as ones you would choose at home. Try to choose foods that will give you something your body needs like protein, vegetables, fruit, or calcium, while avoiding refined carbohydrates, unhealthy fats, and fried foods.

You don't have to eat a "square meal" when you eat out as long as you eat well the rest of the day. If your fast-food restaurant offers a healthy protein and a vegetable, like grilled chicken and salad, but only offers refined carbohydrates, plastic-like artificial cheese, and whole milk, skip the carbs and calcium at that meal.

The three cardinal rules of fast-food dining will help you eat better when fast food is your only option.

1. The first rule of eating out is *drink water*. Avoid sweetened drinks and their empty calories. Unless you really need a dose of caffeine, avoid caffeinated tea and sodas too. Diet soft drinks contain artificial sweeteners with uncertain effects on the body. In addition, all carbonated beverages, whether sweetened or not, can cause calcium loss from the bone, which sets you up for osteoporosis, and weaken your tooth enamel, which sets you up for cavities. Your best bet is to drink water. You will save money, and feel less pressured to buy a combo meal that comes with fries.

2. The second rule, as you may have guessed, is *replace the fries and chips*. They pack plenty of calories and lack any nutritional benefits. Some fast-food restaurants are now offering fruit, side salads, yogurt, and other vegetable options. Decide which ones, if any, suit your taste.

3. The third rule is to *avoid refined carbohydrates*. If your fast-food restaurant doesn't offer any whole-grain options, skip the bread. Make protein and vegetables the emphasis of your fast-food meal.

*In the time it takes to drive to a fast-food joint, you could probably go to a grocery store and pick up fruit, yogurt, nuts, whole-grain bread, granola, or even a salad if the store has a salad bar.*

Avoiding fast-food restaurants altogether is the best choice. Recent studies have linked the number of fast-food chains in an area to the rate of obesity in that community. In the time it takes to drive to a fast-food joint, you could probably go to a grocery store and pick up fruit, yogurt, nuts, whole-grain bread, granola, or even a salad if the store has a salad bar. You'll probably save money and eat better.

## Careful with Buffets

Restaurants with all-you-can-eat buffets can also be quick and healthy, if you don't overdo it; but they can also be one of the biggest dietary mistakes too. Don't go into a buffet restaurant without a plan. If the restaurant has great salads, stick with them. Many buffets have a large variety of vegetables too. Fill your plate with vegetables, leaving up to one-quarter of your plate for lean protein. Avoid the fried foods entirely. Also avoid the empty carbohydrates like rolls, muffins, breaded meats, macaroni and cheese, white pasta, white potatoes, and desserts unless they are the best things on the bar. Then pick your indulgence. Just keep the portion size moderate.

Plan on making no more than two trips. Load your plate with healthy vegetables and lean protein the first trip, then have an indulgence or two on your second trip. You'll be less likely to overindulge if you have already calmed your appetite with your veggies.

*Sometimes a bite or two of a decadent food can be as satisfying as a larger serving.*

If you have the will power to resist dessert, then more power to you! If not, try to select just one and limit the portion size. Sometimes a bite or two of a decadent food can be as satisfying as a larger serving. If any part of the meal is not as tasty as it looked, don't feel obliged to eat it. Leave it on your plate.

Being very familiar with the items on a buffet can help you keep your eating in check. You won't be tempted by every item if you know that certain ones just aren't that tasty or give you indigestion. If you still pig out every time you go to a buffet, then don't go.

*If any part of the meal is not as tasty as it looked, don't feel obliged to eat it. Leave it on your plate.*

# Menu Choices

Chain restaurants that serve from a menu frequently offer healthy eating choices these days. However, their idea of healthy food and your idea of healthy food might not be the same thing. Many restaurants are still stuck in the low-fat era, where refined carbohydrates, skimpy servings of vegetables, and sugary desserts are on the health food menu as long as they contain less than 30 percent fat.

Newer menus boast high-protein-no-carb dishes that are dripping with saturated fat. Choose your meal carefully to include foods that your body needs. Whole-grain dishes are hard to come by. White rice, white pasta, white potatoes, and white breads are the norm. When you plan to eat out, it's a good idea to get your whole grains in at another meal and focus on the healthy foods that restaurants do serve: protein and veggies.

Don't hesitate to ask your waiter or chef for details about the meal you've ordered. Restaurants can often adjust a dish to suit your nutritional needs. However, when you have the opportunity to dine at a fine restaurant, you're likely there to indulge or to celebrate. As long as you don't indulge that often, choose a dish you like and don't pick it apart nutritionally. Enjoy your meal and stop when satisfied. Don't be embarrassed to ask for a doggie bag.

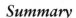

## *Summary*

You'll eat a healthier diet if you eat at home most of the time, but when you do eat out, consider it a treat. You didn't have to shop, cook, or most importantly, clean up. Take a moment to appreciate this. Most of all, eat slowly and enjoy your food. Remember the three cardinal rules of eating out:

1. Drink water, not sweetened or carbonated beverages.
2. Skip the fries and chips.
3. Avoid refined carbohydrates. Choose lean proteins and veggies instead.

# CHAPTER 16

# How to Achieve Permanent Weight Loss

O nce you and your doctor have determined that you're overweight, it's time to set a reasonable weight loss goal for yourself. Measure your height and use the BMI chart (page 62) to determine what weight range would give you a healthy BMI between nineteen and twenty-four.

Next, consider when was the last time (if ever in your adult life) your weight was in that range. If your weight gain occurred over a relatively short period of time, less than five years, expect that you may take half as long to lose the excess weight as you did to put it on. While initial weight loss may be fairly rapid, those who have always been overweight can reasonably expect to lose fifteen to thirty pounds a year, not more.

Dieting can certainly take weight off faster, but the weight doesn't generally stay off. Rebound weight gain often exceeds the original weight loss. Rapidly losing and regaining weight is very stressful to the body, especially if you end up weighing more than you did before dieting. Unless you're very obese and your doctor considers weight loss to be urgent, gradual weight loss is easier and better for you.

It's important to start with reasonable goals. Losing weight slowly while making lifestyle changes is more likely to end up as permanent weight loss. Losing more than about a pound a week is most likely to be a temporary weight loss. Healthy weight loss is slow and steady and does not involve starvation, deprivation, or excessive exercise.

*Dieting can certainly take weight off faster, but the weight doesn't generally stay off. Rebound weight gain often exceeds the original weight loss.*

*Healthy weight loss is slow and steady and does not involve starvation, deprivation, or excessive exercise.*

## How Do I Get Started Losing Weight?

It's useful to try to figure out why you're overweight in the first place. Some of us are born with a big appetite and a love of food. If you fall into this category, there are three major things that will help you lose weight.

- ∾ First, you must *reduce your intake of calorie-dense foods* like sweetened beverages, fried foods, whole-fat dairy products, creamy sauces, sweets, and fatty meats.
- ∾ Secondly, you must adjust your *portion size*. When you serve your plate, reduce the portion of carbohydrates you eat by one half. Reduce meats by one third. Try to eat large portions of fruits and vegetables. Visual tricks like using smaller cups and plates actually work. Only eat one serving. Refrigerate the leftovers or package them for tomorrow's lunch before sitting down to your meal so you won't be tempted by seconds. This trick works at restaurants too. Just ask the waiter to bring a to-go box with the entree. Pack half away before you start to eat. Remember you don't have to clean your plate.
- ∾ Thirdly, you must *find a focus other than food*. If you associate watching TV with snacking, find another evening activity most nights. If you get magazines filled with tempting food, read something else for a change. If spending time with your friends means a trip to a coffee shop for mochas or happy hour with a drink or two, suggest meeting for a walk or at a dance club instead. Start new habits. Take a tai chi or art class in the evening instead of watching TV. If stress makes you seek comfort in food, seek support for yourself emotionally. Practice yoga or meditation, join a support group or see a therapist. You owe it to yourself. Everyone needs a cheerleader.

## "I Avoid Fattening Foods Most of the Time, but I'm Still Gaining Weight: What's Going On?"

You might be eating too much of a good thing. Some overweight people eat healthy types of foods but have lost their *ability to sense satiety*. Many become used to eating until full or even stuffed rather than just satisfied. If you frequently have heartburn or indigestion after a meal, you're probably overeating. (Be sure to tell your doctor if you have frequent indigestion or heartburn.) Eating slowly and mindfully is key to regaining the ability to stop when satisfied.

Keeping a diet journal as described in this book (page 4) is a very important step.

- First, notice how often you stop eating when satisfied. At which meals or snacks do you tend to eat until full? Do you eat past the point of satisfaction because you eat too quickly? If so, slow down. Chew each bite. Think about and enjoy your food.
- Do you wait until you're starved to eat? Snack before you get too hungry.
- Do you go back to the kitchen and graze even if you're not hungry? Find another activity to occupy your time. Also, consider that your munchies could be caused by an unfilled nutritional need. Be sure to eat plenty of fruits, vegetables, whole grains, protein, and healthy fats and take a multivitamin.

Some people have *delayed satiety*. If you often eat until you're satisfied only to feel unpleasantly full several minutes later, you need to eat more slowly and take smaller portions. Stop eating just before you're satisfied. Wait twenty to thirty minutes. If you're still hungry, you can always have a snack. You'll have to become adept at visually judging your portion size from experience in order to avoid overeating.

## "I Don't Eat More than My Skinny Friends Do: Why Have I Gained Weight?"

While some overweight people's love of food makes it obvious why they're overweight, other overweight folks really don't seem to eat very differently than thin folks. This is especially true for people who have gradually put on weight over a period of many years. Many middle-aged Americans find they've gained so many inches around the middle that they couldn't possibly fit into the clothes they wore in their twenties, but have trouble figuring out how all those extra pounds got there.

The truth is that it takes very few excess calories or a slight decrease in activity level to cause a significant weight gain over a ten-year period. In fact, if a woman in her thirties finds herself weighing thirty pounds more than she did in her twenties, her weight gain may have been due to a very small daily excess in calories. A thirty-pound weight gain (a barely noticeable three pounds a year) would result from eating just thirty extra calories a day.

*It takes very few excess calories or a slight decrease in activity level to cause a significant weight gain over a ten-year period.*

That's the cream in your coffee, six chocolate chips, six peanuts, or a few sips of wine.

A thirty-pound weight gain could also come from a small change in activity level. Perhaps she started going to the gym three times a week instead of four, or she traded her more active waitressing job for the job of hostess. Those thirty extra calories a day that weren't burned as exercise gradually added up to thirty-extra pounds over the past ten years. If she were to stop eating those extra thirty calories a day, her weight gain would stop.

If your weight gain has been more rapid, you would need to decrease your calories more. Using the same woman in the example above, if she wanted to slim down, she would have to *both* eliminate the extra calories that are causing her to gain weight and eliminate additional calories to create an energy deficit that would allow her to burn stored fat for energy. This is best accomplished both by eating fewer calories *and* by burning more calories through exercising.

If this woman were to eat just sixty fewer calories or burn just sixty more calories a day (a very small sacrifice), she would lose her thirty extra pounds. Unfortunately it would take her ten years to do it. Most people are not willing to wait that long.

Eating 130 fewer calories or burning 130 more calories a day (that's skipping a twelve-ounce soda, a chunk of cheese, or a couple chocolate chip cookies, or walking for thirty minutes every day) will get her a thirty-pound weight loss in three years. This would be a very safe and attainable weight loss that is likely to result in permanent weight loss. However, most people want quicker results.

If she were to eat 330 fewer calories a day (that's skipping one cup of ice cream, or half of a large order of fries, or just substituting a bowl of oatmeal for a bagel with cream cheese) or burn 330 more calories a day (running thirty minutes or walking briskly for an hour each day), she would lose the thirty pounds in one year.

Ideally she would make some sustainable diet changes *and* increase her exercise if she weren't already exercising most days. For example, if she started walking forty-five minutes five days a week and started drinking water instead of soda, she could lose thirty pounds in a year.

While these relatively small changes can result in a substantial thirty-pound weight loss over a year's time, weight loss will seem slow at less than a pound a week. Therefore, it's wise to avoid weighing yourself more than once every one or two months unless you actually feel that your clothes are getting tighter. Simply burning more calories than you eat will result in the weight loss you need.

# Why Is It So Hard for Some Folks to Lose Weight and Keep It Off?

Everyone has his or her own unique metabolic and genetic idiosyncrasies. Some people's genes enable them to lose weight or maintain a healthy weight more easily than others. If you are not endowed with a set of those genes, don't despair. You can lose weight, but you must accept that you'll have to work at it. It's difficult and unfair to be a small person or have a slow metabolism in a super-sized world. Accept that your portions will not be as big as some other people's. The good news is that we now know how to use your body's own hormones to help you lose weight.

# "If Hormones Can Help Me Lose Weight, Can I Just Take a Hormone Pill?"

The hormones involved in satiety, weight loss, and weight gain are extremely complex. That's why there's no such thing as a diet pill that will control appetite without serious side effects. Each of our body's hormones are intricately intertwined to the point that we could not begin to make a safe and effective diet drug that can do for us what proper nutrition and exercise can do. We can, however, use what we do know about satiety hormones to our advantage.

It's important to know that all body fat is not alike. Notice that people tend to have one of two basic body types. Some people tend to accumulate more fat around their butt and thighs (subcutaneous or sub-Q fat). These people are often called "pear" body types. Others accumulate more fat in their belly (abdominal fat), even if their arms and legs remain relatively thin. These people are termed "apples".

We all have some sub-Q fat and some belly fat, but where you tend to put most of the excess fat you carry predicts your likelihood of developing cancer, heart disease, diabetes, and obesity.

Recently, researchers have discovered that our fat cells are not passive storage cells, but virtual hormone factories, churning out hormones that influence satiety, insulin resistance, blood pressure, inflammation, and our immune system.

## Do Sub-Q Fat Cells and Belly Fat Cells Produce the Same Hormones?

No. If you happen to be a pear, consider yourself lucky. You have more sub-Q fat than belly fat. That means your metabolism is naturally working to help you maintain normal weight. Our sub-Q fat cells produce our weight loss ally, adiponectin in abundance. This hormone helps us burn body fat for energy and ward off insulin resistance and diabetes.

Our sub-Q fat cells are also capable of producing "satiety hormones" like leptin. Those lovely dimpled waves of cellulite actually send chemical messages that say, "Stop eating! You have stored enough fat." These satiety hormones make us feel satisfied when we have had enough food. If you pay attention to your body and stop when satisfied, you will maintain normal weight. However, once you start eating past the satisfaction point and gaining fat, your body becomes resistant to satiety signals.

If you happen to be an apple, you have some sub-Q fat, but most of your excess fat tends to be stored as belly fat. Belly fat is a different type of fat altogether. While it does produce some satiety hormones, it doesn't produce nearly as much as the sub-Q fat does. Belly fat is a good thing to have around if food is in short supply, and you need to conserve energy between infrequent meals. But here in the land of plenty, conserved fat cells plus abundant food all too often equals obesity. Not only do these stubborn fat cells skimp on producing satiety hormones; but they also produce other hormones that promote high blood pressure, insulin resistance, cancer, and diabetes.

## Is There Any Hope for Apples? Are Apples Always Apples and Pears Always Pears?

A thin apple's metabolism is not much different from that of a thin pear. Neither have much belly fat. It's only after they start to put on *excess* poundage that they are very different. While you are born with a tendency to be either an apple or a pear, your diet, exercise, and lifestyle will determine whether you remain an apple or a pear.

Even pears put on excess belly fat if they eat a diet high in saturated fat, eat lots of high GL foods, go too long between meals or skip meals, or if they have a lot of stress in their lives. Conversely, apples and pears alike who eat regular meals and snacks without getting too hungry in between, eat a diet low in saturated fat and high in fruits, vegetables, and whole grains, and limit stress keep their belly fat to a minimum.

---

### Savvy Eating Tip: Belly Fat

Habits that promote storage of belly fat:

- Diet high in saturated fat
- Eating lots of high GL foods
- Going too long between meals or skipping meals
- Stress

---

# Can Skipping Meals Help Me Lose Weight?

Skipping meals will not help you lose weight. The importance of avoiding getting too hungry cannot be over stressed. When you go too long between meals or skip meals your body produces more of the *anti*-satiety hormone, ghrelin. Ghrelin makes you feel hungry. Eating a meal, especially a meal that includes carbohydrates, is the only way to decrease that anti-satiety hormone. This is one of the many reasons that you need carbohydrates in your diet. Carbohydrates inhibit ghrelin more than protein or fat and give you a feeling of satiety that helps you push away from the table rather than overeating.

*The importance of avoiding getting too hungry cannot be over stressed.*

You can choose to ignore hunger as many dieters do, but your body continues to make ghrelin. You may even get used to the feeling of hunger. Many breakfast skippers say they don't even feel hungry in the morning. However, when you finally do eat again, it feels so good that it's often difficult to stop. It takes longer for satiety to set in. People who skip meals, especially breakfast, tend to more than make up for the calories they didn't eat at the skipped meal by overeating at the next meal.

---

### Savvy Eating Tip: Staying Satisfied

Carbohydrates give you *immediate satisfaction* that enables you to stop eating before you get full. Fats and proteins give you *long-lasting satisfaction* that keeps you from getting the munchies. Fat, protein, and carbohydrates are all necessary for a healthy diet. Try to get all three food types at every meal and most snacks.

Unfortunately, that's not all the harm starving yourself does. Meal skippers tend to develop more belly fat than those who eat regular meals, making weight loss harder in the long run.

*Meal skippers tend to develop more belly fat than those who eat regular meals, making weight loss harder in the long run.*

While there's no doubt that frequently putting your body into starvation mode can actually prevent you from losing the weight you need to lose, eating overly large meals is just as harmful. As discussed earlier, when you eat carbohydrates, your blood sugar goes up and your body releases insulin to bring down the high blood sugar and to store energy in fat cells. The more carbohydrates you eat in a given meal, the more insulin you make. When your blood sugar and insulin rise very high, like after eating a high GL food or after eating a large amount of any carbohydrate, your body makes the hormone resistin. Resistin causes you to be more insulin resistant (like type 2 diabetics) and actually causes more belly fat cells to be made. Those who want to avoid obesity and diabetes need to avoid large meals and high GL foods.

## Eat Small Meals No More than Four Hours Apart

The bottom line is that you need to eat small meals and snacks no more than four hours apart (except while you are sleeping). Never skip meals, especially breakfast. Avoid eating a large number of calories at one time, especially if you're eating carbohydrates. In practical terms, that means limiting each meal (including supper) to one-quarter of your daily calorie needs. For most people, that means no single meal should contain more than about 600 calories at a given time. If you choose to eat dessert, it's a good idea to eat it as a separate snack rather than part of a huge meal.

*The bottom line is that you need to eat small meals and snacks no more than four hours apart (except while you are sleeping). Never skip meals, especially breakfast.*

*If you choose to eat dessert, it's a good idea to eat it as a separate snack rather than part of a huge meal.*

Certainly, most people need more than the 1,800 calories a day that three 600-calorie meals would provide. Small snacks will provide the remaining calories. Active people who need more than 2,000 calories a day need to eat more than three meals a day to supply the calories they need without eating too much at any given meal.

# Could I Have a Hormone Problem that Makes Me Gain Weight?

Metabolic disorders that cause weight gain do exist, but are not the usual cause. Metabolic problems like hypothyroidism usually come with other symptoms like constipation, cold intolerance, and fatigue, or growth failure in children. If you feel that you have symptoms of a metabolic problem, don't hesitate to consult your doctor, but keep in mind that the overwhelming majority of overweight people are overweight because of their eating and exercise habits.

Once you have reached your weight loss goal, you'll remain on the same healthy diet as described in this book. Because you'll be following hunger cues, you will not continue to lose weight; instead you'll begin the process of maintaining a healthy weight. Infrequent measurement of your weight and paying attention to the tightness of your waistband is all that's necessary to make sure your weight doesn't start to creep up again. If you start to regain weight, or if you hit a plateau in weight loss, it's time to do another self-evaluation with a food journal as described in chapter 7.

Small, consistent, every day changes are what will result in attaining and maintaining a healthy weight. Small to moderate changes that you are able to make consistently will result in permanent weight loss. Grand efforts to make dramatic changes in your eating habits are difficult to sustain. If you drop from eating 2,200 calories a day to 1,500 and start exercising all at once, your body will cry out for food. When you experience hunger and ignore it, you're causing a whole cascade of hormones that will work to prevent you from losing weight.

*Small to moderate changes that you are able to make consistently will result in permanent weight loss.*

People with lots of will power can lose weight temporarily by starving themselves, but it's rare to keep it off. Your hormones will work against you if you eat high GL foods and don't give your body the vitamins, minerals, fat, and protein it needs. Weight loss will be a constant battle.

However, if you avoid sweetened drinks, switch to whole grains, eat more fruits and vegetables, and eat modest portions of protein and fat at each meal, you will be using your body's natural hormonal check and balance system to work with you to cause weight loss. Gradual changes will prevent your body from feeling like it's starving. Eating satisfying foods and small meals will allow you to eat fewer calories without feeling too hungry.

Gradually trimming down portion size while switching to high nutrient density foods will make weight loss easier. Mindful eating at the table, not in front of the TV, will help you eat less and enjoy more. While willpower is necessary to help you eat the right kinds of foods most of the time, you won't be miserable and starving while you do it. It's what you choose nine times out of ten that counts.

# Here Today, Gone Tomorrow:
# Why Fad Diets Have a Short Shelf Life

As the percentage of overweight people in our society increases, so does the number of fad diets. Unfortunately, extreme and quick fix diets that promise fast results but ignore the basic principles of good nutrition are a prescription for disaster. Some fad diets, like the low-fat high-carb diet, and diets that emphasize eating limited types of food, are unsatisfying and hard to stick to. These diets usually lead to only temporary weight loss followed by rebound weight gain. This yo-yo pattern is more detrimental to good health than maintaining a steady, albeit excessive weight.

*Extreme and quick fix diets that promise fast results but ignore the basic principles of good nutrition are a prescription for disaster.*

Liquid diets, where one or more meals a day are replaced by a liquid dietary supplement, fit into the yo-yo category. These diets only work while you are continuing to replace a meal with a shake, and do nothing to promote healthy eating habits. The one exception to this rule is for the person who does not eat breakfast. Having a liquid supplement for breakfast when the alternative is skipping breakfast is a reasonable and sustainable way to improve ones health. Breakfast is an extremely important meal and should never be skipped. Solid foods like fruits, whole grains, and lean proteins are better choices, but a liquid supplement is better than nothing.

Diet plans that involve the support of dietitians and other dieters are often helpful, but buying prepared food from the system can be expensive and the quality of the meals are usually inferior to what you can make at home. The purchased meals are often high in refined carbohydrates and low in fruits and vegetables. Many plans still require you to do the work of preparing fruits and vegetables (the foods most Americans are least likely to prepare on their own).

Extremely low-carb, high-protein diets have become very popular. Unfortunately, many of these diets condone all proteins, regardless of their saturated fat content, and shun all carbohydrates, regardless of their nutritional value, in order to throw the metabolism into a chemical imbalance that supports fat loss. These diets are risky. There is some risk of dehydration early in the diet, even in healthy people, but most of the risk occurs down the road.

Although there is no research to prove the long-term risks and benefits of these diets, there is theoretical risk of kidney damage, liver damage, and osteoporosis later in life. The most important late side effects are the increased risk of cardiovascular disease and cancers that are common in those who do not eat a diet rich in fruits, vegetables, and whole grains. These complications of the low-carb, high-protein diet aren't likely to develop for many years, so dieters feel complacent about the risks and revel in eating plates of bacon while losing weight. Most of those who initially lose weight regain it when they start eating more carbohydrates. Let's face it, carbs are hard to resist.

Diets that stress the importance of eating a moderate amount of protein and fewer carbohydrates are definitely headed in the right direction. However, they often fall short of making all the recommendations necessary to have a healthy diet. Avoiding empty carbs is key in maintaining healthy weight, but subsisting on large amounts of animal fats and proteins in this day and age is risky.

Animals raised for meat in this country are generally grain-fed. "Grain-fed" is a euphemism for an unnatural and unhealthy animal diet. Grain-fed animals' meat is of poorer nutritional quality than animals raised on natural diets. Healthy human populations, like the Eskimo, who live on an almost exclusively meat diet have done well because the meat they eat is primarily raised on a natural diet. You, too, could probably live on an almost exclusively meat diet if you chose to eat wild fish, grass-fed bison, and truly free-range chicken. However, when these types of animal proteins are available, they tend to be expensive. Most people simply can't afford to eat this way.

A healthy diet does include plenty of proteins and fats, but you must choose your sources of fats and proteins with great care. Animal proteins, even red meat, are healthy choices if they were raised naturally. If you eat commercial grain-fed animals, you should consider eating less animal protein and more protein from other sources. If you do eat naturally fed animal products, then feel free to follow a low-carb diet as long as you include five to thirteen servings a day of fruits and vegetables. It's of major importance to eat plenty of fruits and vegetables with any diet. Fruits and veggies are full of antioxidants that we need to live in modern society. Primitive man did not breathe pollution-filled air and have the exposures that we do to toxic chemicals; nor did he live as long as we do. All of these things make modern man require more antioxidants. Unfortunately, the over-farmed soil of our country is depleted of many of the nutrients that it once had. Commercially farmed produce has fewer nutrients than naturally farmed produce did a century ago. So we have more reason than ever to eat more fruits and vegetables. Remember, no diet is a healthy diet if it does not include lots of produce.

> *Commercially farmed produce has fewer nutrients than naturally farmed produce did a century ago. So we have more reason than ever to eat more fruits and vegetables.*

The best diet for losing weight is one that can be maintained for the rest of your life, but there are times when fad diets can be useful temporarily (for example, phase one of most low-carb diets). If you're very overweight and very dependent on carbohydrates, especially sweets, an extremely low-carb diet will probably help you get started losing the weight you need to lose. Initial weight loss is usually rapid (more than one to two pounds a week), which can be of psychological benefit. But the main reason to try one of these diets is that they help you break an addiction to sweets and empty carbohydrates. However, an extremely low-carb diet should only be started under the advice and guidance of your doctor.

Fad diets usually fail because they are too one-sided. Eating well involves both avoiding foods such as trans fats and refined carbohydrates that harm our bodies and working to include foods such as fruits, vegetables, healthy oils, and whole grains that benefit our bodies. Eating satisfying nutritious food helps you limit caloric intake without starving. Diets that aim to restrict food choices without taking positive action to include the whole foods our bodies need are bound to fail.

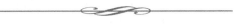

## Summary

For permanent weight loss,

1. Avoid calorie dense foods like sweetened drinks, sweets, refined carbohydrates, fried foods, fatty meats, and full-fat dairy products whenever possible.
2. Decrease portion size, especially for carbohydrates, but don't try to eliminate carbohydrates, they're good for you.
3. Eat more fruits and vegetables.
4. Find a focus other than food.
5. Set reasonable weight loss goals. Understand that quick fixes don't last and can even make it more difficult to lose weight in the future.

6. Use your own hormones to help you lose weight while feeling satisfied. Eat frequent small meals (at least every four hours during the day) with fruits or vegetables, healthy fats, and lean protein at each meal.
7. Never skip meals or let yourself stay hungry for long. You will send hormone messages to your body that will pack on belly fat and prevent you from losing weight.
8. Do vigorous exercise most days.
9. Avoid fad diets.

# CHAPTER 17

# Stocking the Pantry

The plethora of good and bad food choices available to us is mind boggling. The average supermarket has dozens of varieties of cereals, several aisles of snack foods, and hundreds of different beverages. Having good food habits you rely on the majority of the time keeps you from being overwhelmed by the choices you face when you enter the grocery store or wonder, "What's for dinner?"

## Being Prepared Makes Savvy Eating Easy

I, by no means, would imply that you should limit variety in your diet, merely limit the number of decisions you make on a regular basis by eliminating poor choices from your list. Once you discover how easy it is to make healthy snacks and soups and bake simple, delicious breads, you'll be able to skip entire aisles at the grocery store and focus on buying fresh whole foods. You'll no longer need a separate baking mix for pancakes, muffins, brownies, breads, and cakes. Your pantry will be well stocked, but less cluttered, and will have everything you need to make healthier, less expensive versions of the foods you like when you want them.

## Take a Good Look at Your Refrigerator

To start limiting excess choices and eating better take a good look at your refrigerator and pantry. You undoubtedly have a few things lurking in there that you'd be better off not eating.

First, check your shelves for items that contain *trans fats*. Most of these things will be shortenings, margarine, snack foods, convenience mixes, baked goods, and other processed foods. You may not expect to find trans fats in whole grain cereals, granola bars, trail mixes, and peanut butter, but they're often there. The breading on fish and chicken nuggets usually contains trans fats too. Check all your labels for words like "partially hydrogenated," which means trans fat.

Either toss the foods that contain trans fats or resolve not to buy them again once they're gone. Then look for brands that don't have trans fats. (They're becoming more available.) Or determine if you can substitute another food you like for the trans-fat-containing food. For example, most chips are fried in partially hydrogenated oil. There are, however, brands that are fried in healthier oils. You could switch to those brands and eat them in moderation (they're still empty calories), or replace your chips with a healthy snack like fruit or nuts. Make changes and substitutions that you can live with over a long period of time without feeling deprived. If you don't like raw carrot sticks, then they're not an acceptable substitute for your favorite chip.

*Make changes and substitutions that you can live with over a long period of time without feeling deprived. If you don't like raw carrot sticks, then they're not an acceptable substitute for your favorite chip.*

Some substitutions will be unnoticeable while others will take some getting used to. For example, most major brands of peanut butter have some trans fats added to preserve freshness. Natural peanut butter is available in most super markets, but it does have a different texture and needs to be stored in the refrigerator to prevent it from becoming rancid after opening. If you eat a lot of peanut butter, the amount of trans fat in major brands is probably significant over time, so natural brands are your best bet. You will probably adjust to the texture (or prefer it) in time. If natural peanut butter is a little hard to spread straight out of the refrigerator, pop it in the microwave for a few seconds first. Most healthy changes involve adjustment rather than sacrifice.

Rid your refrigerator of any milk that is not skim milk. It's true that skim milk is noticeably different from whole milk; it's thinner and less creamy. But taking ten grams of saturated fat (the amount found in two glasses of whole milk) out of your diet is worth making the adjustment.

The next things to search for in your pantry are refined carbohydrates. Sugar, quick bread and cake mixes, candy, sweet or refined cereals, sodas, and cookies are the most obvious sources; but white breads, white pastas, white rice, chips, and pretzels are all empty calories that could be replaced by healthier foods too. If the first ingredient in a bread, cereal, or snack food is not a whole grain, replace the food with one that is whole grain. Substitute 100 percent (preferably stone–ground) whole-grain bread for white or brown bread that does not list whole wheat or other whole grains as the first ingredient. (Remember, if the label says "wheat flour" rather than *whole*-wheat flour" it's not whole grain.) Substitute whole-grain pasta for white pasta; brown rice for white rice. Even a high-fiber breakfast cereal might not be whole grain and could contain added sugar, salt, and preservatives. Look for cereals with fewer than ten grams of sugar per serving. Try substituting oatmeal for cereals with ingredients you can't pronounce. Avoid fried foods like tortilla chips even if they are whole grain.

No need to waste your money on sodas, juices, and sweetened drinks. Water is the only beverage that you need to drink. Skim milk is one of the best sources of calcium and lean protein and is a healthy addition to your diet if you have no trouble digesting it. Otherwise consider an unsweetened soy beverage to replace milk. All other beverages are optional. Don't waste your money if you can do without them.

## Stock Up on Healthy Foods

Once you've purged your pantry of foods you don't need, you need to fill your pantry, refrigerator, and freezer with whole grains, healthy fats, fruits, vegetables, lean meats, fish, nuts, and spices. Having a well-stocked pantry will make cooking and eating healthy meals at home simple.

To make sure you have enough healthy fats in your diet, keep canola oil, olive oil, ground flax seeds, and a variety of nuts and peanut butter on hand. Buy fresh fish the day you plan to use it, or keep frozen fish filets in the freezer.

Buy quality brands of whole-grain flours, whole-grain pastas, oats, brown rice, and other grains. Experiment with less common grains like quinoa, barley, millet, and amaranth and keep your favorites on hand. Try several brands of whole-grain bread and decide which ones you like best and keep those in your pantry or freezer.

Keep lots of frozen vegetables and fruits as well as refrigerated root vegetables like onions, garlic, sweet potatoes, and carrots on hand so you can put together a healthy meal even if you haven't been to the grocery store in a few days. Canned tomato paste, tomato sauce, and beans are great pantry staples. Organic varieties tend to contain less salt than other brands. Frozen berries make a great addition to oatmeal or yogurt. Frozen peas and spinach are almost as good as fresh in some dishes.

---

### Savvy Eating Tip: Staying the Course

Enthusiasm for healthy eating waxes and wanes. Re-read this book from time to time to keep inspired, but don't become overly focused on food. You will not necessarily be able to or want to follow all the recommendations in this book, but each improvement you are able to make and maintain over your lifetime will have significant health benefits.

Spices are full of antioxidants as well as flavor. Keep chili powder, garlic powder, curry spices, cumin, coriander, oregano, rosemary, thyme, cinnamon, ginger, allspice, and other spices on your shelf.

When you start to eat more fruits and vegetables, you may find it necessary to go to the grocery store more than once a week. Even this task can be streamlined if you make one weekly trip to get non-perishable staples *and* fresh fruits, vegetables and fish, and the second trip later in the week for fresh items only. Limiting your shopping to the outer aisles of the store will limit excess choices and make the second trip quicker and more efficient. (Prepackaged foods tend to be in the central isles of the store, while fresh produce, dairy products, and fish tend to be on the outer aisles.) Alternatively, shop once a week at the grocery store and later in the week at the local farmer's market or co-op to get fresh seasonal produce.

The pleasant surprise is that keeping a well-stocked, healthy pantry will save you money. Even though some healthy foods are pricey, whole foods are generally less expensive than processed prepackaged foods, convenience foods, and eating out. After going through a phase of experimentation and adjustment involving different and healthier foods, you'll find that choosing healthy foods will become easier. The knowledge of nutrition you've gained reading this book will help you easily eliminate many poor food choices. Ask yourself, "How will this food benefit my body?" before you eat it. Appreciate what good it does for your body. You'll feel the temptation to indulge in foods that aren't good for your body ebb away.

*Keeping a well-stocked, healthy pantry will save you money.*

However, when you decide to eat unhealthy food on occasion, appreciate it for the pleasure it gives you at that moment rather than feeling guilt. Eating well most of the time affords you the luxury of indulgence now and then. This is especially important at times of celebration. Avoid sweets most of the time, but don't feel you can't eat birthday cake. (Unless, of course, you celebrate birthdays with an unusually large number of people.) Use the nine out of ten rule if you're not sure how much indulgence is too much. If you exhibit good habits, such as eating five to nine fruits and veggies a day, getting your daily omega-3s, eating whole grains, eating two or fewer empty carbs a day—nine times out of ten, it's unlikely you will have anything to worry about, especially if you maintain a stable healthy weight.

*However, when you decide to eat unhealthy food on occasion, appreciate it for the pleasure it gives you at that moment rather than feeling guilt. Eating well most of the time affords you the luxury of indulgence now and then.*

Keep in mind that any food you eat three or more times a week is not an occasional indulgence; it's a staple. There is no such thing as a perfect diet. A wise and happy person will strive for a diet that is not perfect, but good enough.

# Start Cooking

Now that you understand the basic principles of good nutrition, it's time to put your nutrition knowledge into practice. The remainder of this book will show you how to take action. First, get more fruits and vegetables into your diet by learning a few easy methods for preparing them at home. Learn to make soups and salads a daily habit. Make several of the healthy soup recipes in this book staples in your diet. The section on salads will provide you with tips on making delicious salads convenient. Eating more soups and salads will take the emphasis off eating large amounts of meat and increase the amount of protein you get from legumes and nuts.

> *There is no such thing as a perfect diet. A wise and happy person will strive for a diet that is not perfect, but good enough.*

Learn easy and versatile cooking methods for almost any vegetable. When veggies are tasty, interesting, and easy to prepare, you'll eat more of them. You will no longer have an excuse for neglecting your daily vegetable needs.

A few basic techniques for fish and chicken will help you put together easy healthy meals without fuss. Learn to prepare fish and poultry then freeze it in convenient and economical ready-to-use packages.

Next, you'll rethink the way you make pasta dishes to include whole-grain pastas and more vegetables. Add whole-grain pilafs, pizzas, and cereals to your food repertoire too. You can learn how to enjoy whole-grain, less-processed baked goods by learning to make them yourself following a few basic recipes and their variations. Then last but not least, learn how

---

### Savvy Eating Tip: Envision Your Goals

Before it becomes your reality, you must envision it. Make a conscious effort to envision yourself and your family as Savvy Eaters. Don't sabotage your efforts to eat well or lose weight with negative images of yourself, your eating habits, or your family's eating habits. Take a moment to imagine yourself and your family eating and enjoying nutritious food together. If you can imagine it, you can do it.

to satisfy sweet cravings with less sugary, whole-grain desserts that use healthy fats in place of butter and trans fats.

Read through the introduction to each section to get an explanation of each technique, then look at the recipes and decide which ones will enrich your diet, tantalize your taste buds, and make your life simpler. Decide which foods to make staples in your diet, focusing on nutrition, taste, and simplicity.

Use the methods and recipes in this book to replace any old habits that do not provide good nutrition, satisfaction, and peace of mind. Remember, no one's diet is perfect. No matter how good your intentions, you will eat some foods that aren't good for your body, and that's OK.

## *Summary*

In order to make Savvy Eating easy for you, use these guidelines.

1. Rid your pantry of trans fats. Stock up on flax seeds, healthy oils, and fish.
2. Replace sweets and refined grain products with whole grains.
3. Don't buy sweet drinks. Skim milk is the only drink you *need* to buy.
4. Stock up on fresh, frozen, and even canned fruits and vegetables.
5. Keep healthy herbs and spices on hand to enhance food flavors and boost nutrition.
6. Streamline your shopping so you can efficiently shop for fresh foods two or more times a week.
7. Learn cooking techniques that make Savvy Eating easy, quick, economical, and delicious.

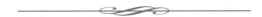

# CHAPTER 18

# What's for Dinner?
# A Thirty-Day Meal Plan

**Y**ou can follow these meal plans exactly and take advantage of the tips for time-saving cooking sessions that help you prepare parts of several meals at a time. Leftovers are often incorporated into the next day's menu to save time and effort. To take advantage of seasonal produce, substitute fruits and vegetables that are in season for the suggested ones whenever you like. Larger families will have to double recipes in order to have leftovers.

## How to Use the Thirty-Day Meal Plan

Many of the meals are designed to go from pantry or freezer to the table in thirty minutes or less. You'll save time by preparing tomorrow's lunch while preparing tonight's supper. No hassle in the morning and you clean up the kitchen only once.

If you don't want to use these meal plans exactly as written, you can use them as guidelines for individual days or meals to help you plan your Savvy Eating. They will help you get five to nine servings of vegetables and fruits, at least two servings of dairy calcium, plenty of whole grains, and healthy proteins and fats every day. Even if you aren't following the plans exactly, take a look at the tips. They'll help you make the most of your time spent in the kitchen.

*If you don't want to use these meal plans exactly as written, you can use them as guidelines for individual days or meals to help you plan your Savvy Eating.*

Notice that the serving size for most of the dishes is not included. This is because this meal plan was created for everyone in your family. There may be some 2,500-calorie appetites as well as some 1,600-calorie appetites. Serving size depends on an individual's needs. The key is to start with a modest portion and eat until satisfied—not stuffed.

If you're trying to lose weight, stick to modest portions of the foods on the meal plan and take small portions of the breads, grains, pastas, and sweets. Add as many additional vegetables and low GL fruits as you wish. Add up to three servings of coffee or unsweetened tea if you like.

*The key is to start with a modest portion and eat until satisfied—not stuffed.*

If your weight is stable and you're an active person, you can add in some extras like beer or wine two to three times a week, desserts (preferably from one of the recipes in this book) or other snacks. A good rule for eating moderately is to have either dessert *or* an alcoholic beverage on any given day, not both. Only indulge in both if you have something to celebrate.

Even if you're at a healthy weight and active, try to limit *empty* carbs to two servings a day most days. There will be some days when you have a pastry for breakfast, fast food for lunch, or take-out pizza and chicken wings for supper. As long as that is the rare exception rather than the rule, don't worry about it. Your diet will not be perfect. If you're planning to celebrate with cake after dinner, cut back on carbohydrates at your other meals that day. Eat healthier carbs the next day.

*If your weight is stable and you're an active person, you can add in some extras like beer or wine two to three times a week, desserts (preferably from one of the recipes in this book) or other snacks.*

You may want to simplify by eating quick-to-fix whole-grain cereal or oatmeal each weekday morning rather than the variety of breakfast choices in the meal plan. If your busy day does not allow for snacks, then eat the morning snack as part of breakfast, and the afternoon snack as part of lunch, or as an after dinner snack (as long as you don't eat right before bedtime).

If you don't have access to a microwave at lunch, you'll have to modify the lunch menus. Soups can often be kept hot enough in a thermos if your lunch hour is not too late. Substitute salads, black bean dip and pita chips, hummus and veggie sandwiches, or peanut butter sandwiches with fruit or raw veggies for hot dishes if you like. You may want to substitute prepackaged soup for homemade, simple salads and prepared dressings for the specific recipes given, and stone-ground tortilla chips for homemade pita chips to save time. Just be sure to read the labels carefully to avoid trans fats, excess salt, and refined grains (Your chip should have visible chunks of corn.) Try Garden of Eatin' blue corn chips and Pacific brand boxed soups.

*A good rule for eating moderately is to have either dessert or an alcoholic beverage on any given day, not both. Only indulge in both if you have something to celebrate.*

Reading the section on preparing poultry and fish in advance will greatly improve your efficiency in the kitchen as well as save you money.

There will be nights when you quickly pull frozen chicken or fish and commercial frozen vegetables out of the freezer for an easy, no-mess supper. There are other times when you will opt for simple preparations. For example, you can just serve plain leftover brown rice on day two rather than preparing Stir Fried Rice or use a prepared seasoning mix or marinade to season meat.

*There will be nights when you quickly pull frozen chicken or fish and commercial frozen vegetables out of the freezer for an easy, no-mess supper.*

Packing your lunch the night before is a huge time saver for those who rush off to school or work in the morning. It also helps those who stay at home limit portion size. Recycled plastic take-out bowls with tight lids and purchased disposable plastic bowls with lids are perfect for packing salads. Just prepare the salad the night before when you are preparing supper. Put the dressing in a zip-top plastic bag. If you don't have any salad dressing prepared, put equal parts olive oil and vinegar in a zip top bag with a shake of mixed dried herbs or garlic powder.

If you're having leftover soup or pasta for lunch, pack them into lunch containers when you put away supper so you just have to take it out of the refrigerator in the morning. Pack single servings of snacks in plastic zip-top bags or recycled plastic containers. This makes healthy snacks convenient and limits portion size.

You'll notice that other than skim milk, there are very few beverages on the menu. Water is always the beverage of choice. Drink plenty of water with each meal and snack as well as throughout the day.

The meal plans include at least two servings of dairy calcium a day. (Sometimes in the form of skim milk or non-fat yogurt, and sometimes incorporated into dishes like **Fruit and Nut Breakfast Pilaf or Protein-Packed Morning Oats.**) You can add another portion of dairy, or just take a multivitamin with calcium daily to get your three servings a day. (Most multivitamins contain about 30 percent of your daily calcium needs. Check the label.)

If you can't tolerate dairy foods, you'll want to substitute protein-containing foods like nuts, peanut butter, or fortified soy products for the milk, yogurt, or cheese. You will also need to take additional calcium supplements if your substitutions don't contain calcium.

Vegetarians can omit the meats in the menu and substitute beans, eggs, nuts, tofu, soy protein, or other protein sources. Many of the meals are already meatless.

Young children can be a challenge when planning meals. If your children are very young, you may need to offer them alternate foods. After nine to twelve months of age, kids do well with soups, chopped meats, cereals, pastas, breads, fruit, and chopped cooked vegetables, but don't do well with salads or raw vegetables. Offering kids fruit instead of salads and raw veggies is one simple solution. You will also want to hold off on nuts until age three when they develop the chewing coordination to handle such dangerous choking hazards. (Peanuts, whole grapes, and hot dogs are among the leading causes of choking among children.) Hard fruits like apples should be peeled and sliced thinly. Grapes should be cut in half or quarters depending on size. Do offer children the same foods you eat whenever possible.

Note: The recipes included in this book are in bold print.

# The Thirty-Day Meal Plan

## DAY: 1

**Breakfast:** Whole-grain toast with peanut butter and 8 ounces skim milk
**Snack:** 1 orange or seasonal fruit
**Lunch: Favorite Winter Salad**
**Snack:** 4 ounces plain non-fat yogurt with 1 teaspoon honey (optional), and 2 tablespoons wheat germ or nuts.
**Supper: Roasted Southwest Chicken Breasts; Roasted Carrots, Sweet Potatoes, Onions, and Brussels Sprouts; Herbed Brown Rice** or plain brown rice; **Roasted Pears**

**Tips:** *The chicken, carrots, sweet potatoes, onions, Brussels sprouts, and pears can be roasted at the same time at 450 degrees for times specified by the roasting chart on page 201. Roast more than you need for tonight and have the leftovers on your salad for lunch. Pack your lunch salad as you clean up after supper.*

## DAY: 2

**Breakfast: Quick Fruit and Nut Breakfast Pilaf**
**Snack:** Apple dipped in peanut butter
**Lunch:** Leftover **Roasted Vegetables and Southwest Chicken** over salad greens with **Quick Vinaigrette**
**Snack:** 8 ounces skim milk with or without 1 tablespoon chocolate milk mix
**Supper: Asian Marinated Broiled Chicken Breasts,** leftover brown rice, **Wilted Spinach with Garlic and Olive Oil,** steamed carrots and snow peas

**Tips:** *While broiling chicken, steam carrots for 10 minutes, add the snow peas to the same pot, then steam for another 5 minutes until they're tender. If you're making homemade hummus and Greek salad for lunch to-*

*morrow, do it while supper is cooking and clean up just once. Substitute commercial hummus and a simple salad if you wish.*

## DAY: 3

**Breakfast:** 2 eggs *or* 1 egg and 2 egg whites scrambled, whole-grain bread toasted with 1 ounce cheddar cheese or 8 ounces skim milk
**Snack:** ½ cup berries or seasonal fruit
**Lunch:** Greek Salad with **Pita Chips and Hummus**
**Snack:** 1 cup non-fat plain yogurt with 1 teaspoon honey (optional) and a peach or seasonal fruit
**Supper:** Quick Beans and Greens Soup with Ham, Pumpkin Oat Bran Muffins, and strawberries

**Tips:** *The soup and muffins cook in about half an hour. Package some for your lunch as you clean up after supper.*

## DAY: 4

**Breakfast:** Protein-Packed Morning Oats
**Snack:** Orange or seasonal fruit
**Lunch:** Leftover **Quick Beans and Greens Soup, Pumpkin Oat Bran Muffin**
**Snack:** Apple or seasonal fruit with 1 ounce cheddar cheese or ½ cup low-fat ricotta cheese with cinnamon for dipping
**Supper:** Southwest Roasted Salmon, Roasted Asparagus, Roasted Carrots, and baked beans

**Tips:** *Roast salmon, asparagus and carrots at the same time at 450 degrees according to the roasting chart. Microwave canned baked beans. Pack tomorrow's lunch.*

## DAY: 5

**Breakfast:** Fluffy Oat Pancakes, 8 ounces skim milk
**Snack:** Strawberries or seasonal fruit
**Lunch:** Favorite Fall Salad with Honey Mustard Vinaigrette
**Snack:** Peanuts
**Supper:** Pasta with Pesto and Veggies, Broiled Chicken Breasts with Italian Marinade, Fruit Smoothie (optional)

**Tips:** *Use fresh chicken breasts or marinated frozen ones that have been partially thawed in the microwave. The pasta with pesto and veggies cooks in one pot. You can use commercial pesto to save a step. Pack tomorrow's lunch as you clean up.*

## DAY: 6

**Breakfast:** Pumpkin Oat Bran Pancakes, 8 ounces skim milk
**Snack:** ½ grapefruit or seasonal fruit
**Lunch:** Leftover **Pasta with Pesto and Veggies** or salad
**Snack:** Non-fat yogurt with honey (optional) and raspberries
**Supper:** Lentils and Brown Rice with Caramelized Onions, Kale with Garlic and Olive Oil, steamed carrots with 1 teaspoon maple syrup (optional)

**Tips:** *This is a simple nutritious supper. Chop veggies and make pita chips and bean dip for tomorrow's lunch while the lentils cook. You can substitute prepared bean dip and pita chips to save time or have leftovers for lunch instead.*

## DAY: 6

**Breakfast:** Protein-Packed Morning Oats
**Snack:** Blueberries or seasonal fruit
**Lunch:** Black Bean Dip with Pita Chips, baby carrots, celery, and red bell pepper strips for dipping
**Snack:** Pistachio nuts and 8 ounces skim milk
**Supper:** Roasted Chicken Breasts with Herbed Marinade, Roasted Acorn Squash with Maple Syrup, steamed broccoli, brown rice

**Tips:** *Start your squash and brown rice first. Even though this is a simple menu, it takes time to cook. While you're roasting tonight's squash, throw in some whole sweet potatoes for tomorrow. You can chop veggies for tomorrow's veggie scramble and Thai salad. Pack your lunch salad while supper cooks.*

## DAY: 7

**Breakfast:** Curried Veggie Scramble and whole-grain bread toasted
**Snack:** Berries with non-fat plain yogurt and 1 teaspoon honey
**Lunch:** Thai Salad or a simple salad
**Snack:** Mixed nuts
**Supper:** Red Beans and Rice, Roasted Sweet Potatoes, Collard Greens with Garlic and Olive Oil, Chocolate Zucchini Cake, and 8 ounces skim milk

**Tips:** ***Red Beans and Rice*** *is simple to prepare. That gives you time to make* ***Chocolate Zucchini Cake*** *(optional). Red beans, rice, and greens are so nutritious and low in calories that you have room in your diet for an indulgence like this whole-grain cake. Remember to pack some beans and rice for lunch.*

## DAY: 8

**Breakfast:** Quick Fruit and Nut Breakfast Pilaf
**Snack:** Orange or other seasonal fruit
**Lunch:** Leftover **Red Beans and Rice** with Monterey Jack cheese, strawberries
**Snack:** Peanuts or roasted soy nuts
**Supper:** Roasted Red Pepper Soup, Broiled Salmon with Asian Marinade, Stir-Fried Rice or plain brown rice, steamed broccoli

**Tips:** *Start the rice about an hour before you want to eat (or use quick-cooking brown rice), then marinate the salmon, then start the soup. Substitute a quality soup like Pacific brand if time is short. Steam broccoli 7 minutes. Pack tomorrow's lunch.*

## DAY: 9

**Breakfast:** 2 eggs or 1 egg and 2 egg whites, whole-grain toast, 8 ounces skim milk
**Snack:** peach or seasonal fruit
**Lunch:** Leftover **Roasted Red Pepper Soup**, grilled cheese sandwich or pita chips with cheese
**Snack:** Apple dipped in peanut butter
**Supper:** Roasted Veggie Pasta with Turkey Sausage, Updated Classic Spinach Salad

**Tips:** *Roast enough veggies to have leftovers for lunch. Pack pita, hummus, and veggies separately so they won't be soggy by lunchtime. Include a knife for spreading the hummus.*

## DAY: 10

**Breakfast:** Fluffy Oat Pancakes, 8 ounces skim milk
**Snack:** Strawberries or seasonal fruit
**Lunch:** ½ whole-grain pita stuffed with **Hummus** and leftover **Roasted Veggies**
**Snack:** Sliced pear dipped in non-fat cream cheese
**Supper:** Roasted Haddock or other white fish with **Herb Marinade**, Roasted Asparagus, Roasted Carrots, Roasted Onions, and Whole-Wheat Blueberry-Raspberry Muffins

**Tips:** *Roast the fish, asparagus, carrots and onions at 450 degrees according to the roasting chart. Mix the muffins while supper cooks. Reduce the heat to 350 and bake the muffins during supper and serve them as dessert. Pack tomorrow's salad.*

## DAY: 11

**Breakfast:** Whole-Wheat Blueberry Raspberry Muffins, 8 ounces skim milk
**Snack:** Watermelon or cantaloupe chunks or seasonal fruit
**Lunch:** Favorite Summer Salad
**Snack:** Peanuts
**Supper:** Tortilla Soup, Quick Refried Bean Burritos, guacamole or avocado slices, Almond Yogurt Cream with Berries

**Tips:** *This great tasting healthy meal requires very little cooking, just assembly of ingredients. Pack tomorrow's lunch. Soak navy beans overnight if you plan to have navy bean soup on day 13.*

## DAY: 12

**Breakfast:** Protein-Packed Morning Oats
**Snack:** Orange or seasonal fruit
**Lunch:** Favorite Winter Salad
**Snack:** Non-fat plain yogurt with 1 teaspoon honey and fresh berries
**Supper:** Roasted Winter Veggie Pasta with Italian Turkey Sausage, Spinach with Garlic and Olive Oil

**Tips:** *Roasting takes over an hour, but once the veggies are in the oven most of the work is done. Just boil and drain pasta and toss with frozen cooked turkey sausage or seasoned turkey (thawed 2–3 minutes in the microwave) to make prep time short. Spinach with Garlic and Olive Oil cooks in just minutes.*

*Navy bean soup calls for many of the same chopped veggies that the pasta does. Chop enough for both and let a pot of soup simmer while you prepare tonight's meal. While you're at it, chop the veggies you need for tomorrow's* **Asian Stir-Fried Rice** *and store the chopped veggies in the refrigerator in an air-tight container. Alternatively, use frozen soup made earlier or a quality canned soup for tomorrow's lunch.*

## DAY: 13

**Breakfast:** Whole-grain toast with peanut or almond butter, 8 ounces skim milk
**Snack:** Peach or seasonal fruit
**Lunch:** Navy Bean Soup, grapes, and whole-grain bread
**Snack:** Raw veggies with Ranch dip
**Supper:** Asian Stir-Fried Rice with Asian Tofu or Broiled Asian Chicken, Asian Slaw, Amaretti Cookies (optional) and 8 ounces skim milk

**Tips:** *Cook the rice an hour before supper and then start the Asian Slaw, and marinate the chicken or tofu. Use packaged shredded cabbage to* *save time if you like. Chop and refrigerate the veggies for tomorrow's* Mexican-Style Scramble *to save time. You can make the* Amaretti Cookies *before of after supper. Pack some soup for tomorrow's lunch.*

## DAY: 14
**Breakfast:** Quick Fruit and Nut Breakfast Pilaf
**Snack:** Orange or seasonal fruit
**Lunch:** Leftover Navy Bean Soup, Pita Chips
**Snack:** Non-fat yogurt with 1 teaspoon honey
**Supper:** Mexican-Style Scramble (egg or tofu) with Updated Classic Spinach Salad with Vidalia Onion Dressing

**Tips:** *This is a quick supper, especially if you cut up the veggies the night before. The Vidalia onion dressing is an extra step but worth it. You can caramelize extra onions to top tomorrow's salad. If you're short on time, skip the caramelized onion and use a prepared dressing tonight and sliced purple onion on tomorrow's salad. Pack tomorrow's salad.*

## DAY: 15
**Breakfast:** Banana Oat Bran Pancakes, 8 ounces skim milk
**Snack:** Grapes
**Lunch:** Green Salad with Caramelized Onions, Bleu Cheese, and Walnuts
**Snack:** Apple slices dipped in peanut butter
**Supper:** Spinach Soup, Roasted Chicken Breasts with Italian Marinade, Roasted Sweet Potatoes, Vanilla Yogurt Cream with berries

**Tips:** *If you're short on time use a packaged soup or one from the freezer. Previously prepared frozen marinated chicken breasts make this meal quick and easy. Roast sweet potatoes and chicken at 450 degrees.*

## DAY: 16
**Breakfast:** Whole-grain cereal with 8 ounces skim milk, topped with chopped walnuts
**Snack:** ½ grapefruit or seasonal fruit
**Lunch:** ½ whole-grain pita stuffed with fat-free cream cheese, 1 ounce grated cheddar cheese, shredded lettuce, bell pepper strips, shredded carrot, and leftover chicken
**Snack:** Oatmeal Spice Cookie
**Supper:** Easy Pasta and Veggies with Tomato Sauce and Turkey Sausage, Greek Salad

**Tip:** *Use frozen cooked turkey sausage thawed in the microwave to save time. Vegetarians substitute white beans. Pack tomorrow's lunch.*

## DAY: 17

**Breakfast:** Protein-Packed Morning Oats
**Snack:** Grapes
**Lunch:** Leftover **Easy Pasta and Veggies with Tomato Sauce,** and/or **Greek Salad**
**Snack:** Peanuts
**Supper:** **Vegetable Barley Soup,** grilled cheese sandwich on whole-grain bread (use olive or canola oil in place of butter), strawberries dipped in chocolate

**Tips:** *Chop veggies for soup and for tomorrow's* **Curried Veggie Scramble.** *Pack a salad or leftovers for lunch.*

## DAY: 18

**Breakfast:** **Curried Veggie Scramble,** 8 ounces skim milk
**Snack:** Berries or seasonal fruit
**Lunch:** **Summer Tossed Salad**
**Snack:** Non-fat yogurt with sliced peaches and 1 teaspoon honey
**Supper:** **White Beans With Pesto and Spinach** over brown rice or toasted whole-grain bread drizzled with olive oil

**Tips:** *This is an easy meal. Pack tomorrow's lunch.*

## DAY: 19

**Breakfast:** Fluffy Oat Pancakes, 8 ounces skim milk
**Snack:** Watermelon chunks or seasonal fruit
**Lunch:** **Favorite Winter Salad**
**Snack:** Toasted almonds, 8 ounces skim milk
**Supper:** **Roasted Salmon with Southwest Dry Rub, Roasted Carrots, Asparagus, and Red Skin Potatoes,** Raspberries

**Tips:** *The salmon and veggies roast at the same time. Put the different veggies on separate sheets of foil so you can easily remove any item that cooks more quickly. Prepare and pack hummus and veggies for tomorrow. You can use leftover roasted veggies in place of the fresh veggies on tomorrow's lunch menu. Use commercial hummus if desired.*

## DAY: 20

**Breakfast:** Protein-Packed Morning Oats
**Snack:** Cantaloupe or seasonal fruit
**Lunch:** Whole-grain pita with **Hummus** and red pepper strips, cucumbers, and shredded carrot

**Snack:** Grapes and almonds
**Supper:** Broiled Chicken with Italian Marinade, Italian Spinach Salad, Flourless Peanut Butter Cookie (optional)

**Tips:** *Tonight's simple supper gets packed away for tomorrow's lunch.*

## DAY: 21
**Breakfast:** Quick Fruit and Nut Breakfast Pilaf
**Snack:** Strawberries or seasonal fruit
**Lunch:** Leftover **Italian Spinach Salad**
**Snack:** Peanuts or **Flourless Peanut Butter Cookie**
**Supper:** Black Bean Chili with shredded cheese and fat-free sour cream over brown rice or with **Pita Chips**, seasonal fruit

**Tips:** *The brown rice takes about an hour to cook (Feel free to substitute quick-cooking brown rice or quinoa), but this meal won't keep you in the kitchen long. Pack leftovers for lunch.*

## DAY: 22
**Breakfast:** Whole-grain cereal with 8 ounces skim milk
**Snack:** Non-fat yogurt with blueberries and 1 teaspoon honey
**Lunch:** Leftover **Black Bean Chili** with shredded cheese and fat-free sour cream
**Snack:** Cashew nuts
**Supper:** Roasted Bell Pepper Pasta with Italian Turkey Sausage, Favorite Summer Salad

**Tips:** *Again tonight's meal packs up easily for tomorrow's lunch.*

## DAY: 23
**Breakfast:** Pumpkin Oat Bran Pancakes, 8 ounces skim milk
**Snack:** Orange or seasonal fruit
**Lunch:** Leftover **Roasted Bell Pepper Pasta** and/or **Favorite Summer Salad**
**Snack:** 8 ounces skim milk with or without chocolate drink mix, strawberries
**Supper:** Broiled Flounder with olive oil, salt, pepper, and lemon juice, steamed broccoli, **Summer Squash with Garlic and Maple Syrup,** toasted almonds and dried apricots dipped in dark chocolate (optional)

**Tips:** *Start squash first, then broil flounder. Steam broccoli 7 minutes. Pack a salad for lunch. Enjoy a no-prep healthy delicious dessert.*

## DAY: 24

**Breakfast:** Fluffy Oat Pancakes, 8 ounces skim milk
**Snack:** Grapes or seasonal fruit
**Lunch:** Favorite Spring Salad
**Snack:** Peanuts and raisins
**Supper:** Roasted Chicken Breasts with Southwest Marinade, Roasted Peppers and Onions, avocado slices, shredded cheese, and shredded lettuce wrapped in a whole-grain tortilla (optional), **Bean and Corn Salad**

**Tips:** *Prepare chicken and veggies for roasting first, then make* **Bean and Corn Salad.** *Pack salad for lunch.*

## DAY: 25

**Breakfast:** Protein-Packed Morning Oats
**Snack:** Cantaloupe or seasonal fruit
**Lunch:** Shredded lettuce salad topped with leftover **Roasted Chicken** and Bean and Corn Salad
**Snack:** Non-fat yogurt with blueberries and 1 teaspoon of honey
**Supper:** Roasted Summer Veggie Pasta, Spinach with Olive Oil and Garlic

**Tips:** *Roasting veggies takes over an hour but not a lot of work. Roast enough for tonight's pasta and tomorrow's pizza. Chop the veggies for tomorrow's* **Garden Veggie Scramble.** *You'll have plenty of time to boil pasta, fix the spinach, and catch up on a good book while it cooks. Pack some leftovers for lunch.*

## DAY: 26

**Breakfast:** Garden Veggie Scramble, 8 ounces skim milk
**Snack:** Orange or seasonal fruit
**Lunch:** Leftover **Roasted Summer Veggie Pasta** or salad
**Snack:** Mixed nuts
**Supper:** Roasted Summer Veggies, Feta, and Pesto on Whole-Wheat Pizza, Green Salad with Caramelized Onions, Bleu Cheese and Walnuts

**Tips:** *This meal can be quick and easy if you use roasted veggies from the day before. You can start the pizza dough in the morning and leave it to rise all day if you wish. Caramelizing onions takes about 15 minutes, but tastes great. Time-saving options would be to roast the onions the night before or use raw onions in the salad. Pack leftovers for lunch.*

## DAY: 27

**Breakfast:** Fruit and Nut Breakfast Pilaf
**Snack:** Non-fat yogurt with peaches and 1 teaspoon honey

**Lunch:** Leftover Pizza and/or Salad

**Snack:** Apple slices dipped in peanut butter

**Supper:** Crustless Spinach Quiche, Curried Carrot Soup, and Whole-Wheat Bread with Flaxseed

*Tips: Prepare the carrot soup while the quiche is baking. Put the bread dough in a bread machine earlier in the day or use commercial whole-grain bread. Pack up lunch.*

## DAY: 28

**Breakfast:** Whole-wheat toast with peanut or almond butter, 8 ounces skim milk

**Snack:** Watermelon or seasonal fruit

**Lunch:** Leftover Curried Carrot Soup, whole-grain bread with fat-free cream cheese and cucumber and bell pepper slices or grilled cheese sandwich

**Snack:** Black Bean Dip with raw veggies and/or Pita Chips

**Supper:** Broiled Salmon with Herb Marinade, Cabbage with Balsamic Vinegar, Mustard, and Raisins, Green Beans with Garlic and Olive Oil, strawberries

*Tips: Get the cabbage started first, then cook the beans while the salmon broils. Make Mandarin Orange Spinach Salad for tomorrow and the next day. Pack some salad for lunch.*

## DAY: 29

**Breakfast:** Pumpkin Oat Bran Pancakes, 8 ounces skim milk

**Snack:** Blueberries or seasonal fruit

**Lunch:** Mandarin Orange Spinach Salad with cubed chicken, tofu, or extra almonds or sunflower seeds

**Snack:** Non-fat yogurt with strawberries and honey

**Supper:** Vegetable Barley Soup, Broiled Chicken Breasts with Italian Marinade over Spinach with Garlic and Olive Oil and whole-grain spaghetti.

*Tips: Use a commercial soup if you need to. Put the cooked pasta into the pan with the finished spinach and toss to coat. Pack soup for lunch.*

## DAY: 30

**Breakfast:** Protein-Packed Morning Oats

**Snack:** 2 clementines or seasonal fruit

**Lunch:** Leftover Vegetable Barley Soup, grilled cheese sandwich or whole-grain crackers and cheese

**Snack:** Peanuts

**Supper:** Red Beans and Rice, leftover Mandarin Orange Spinach Salad, Oatmeal Spice Cookies (optional)

**Tips:** Red Beans and Rice *is an easy dish to fix, and the salad is already made, so you have time to make cookies if you like.*

# CHAPTER 19

# Eating Your Veggies

## *Soups*

oups are the food staples of many cultures for good reason. Few foods are so healthy and satisfying. They're an excellent way to include more vegetables in your diet because they usually contain a variety of different types of vegetables in their most digestible form (boiled). Because the cooking liquid or the broth is eaten along with the soup's vegetables, soup retains many of the nutrients that are normally lost when the cooking liquid is discarded.

Many hearty soups also contain a protein source like beans or meat making them a one-dish meal. When you make soup, the flavorful combinations of individual ingredients meld into a dish that is much more delicious and satisfying than its component parts. Soups can be simple and homespun or spectacular enough to be served at the finest restaurants. Soup is one of the few comfort foods with great health benefits.

*Because the cooking liquid or the broth is eaten along with the soup's vegetables, soup retains many of the nutrients that are normally lost when the cooking liquid is discarded.*

My guess is that those who don't love soup have never had *good* soup. By this I mean soup that didn't come from a can. Canned chicken noodle soups, for example, are often little more than salt water with a few added chemicals. Often, canned soup's lack of flavor is only rivaled by its lack of nutritional benefits as compared to homemade soup.

Manufacturers often cut corners by using lower quality ingredients, then make up for the lack of taste by adding lots of salt. They also add relatively few vegetables. What's more, canned soup often just tastes canned.

That said, when time is short canned soup is often a better choice than fast food, but only if you choose the can carefully. Choose canned soups that have vegetables as the first ingredients, less than 500 mg of sodium per serving, and no additives that you can't pronounce.

*Soup is one of the few comfort foods with great health benefits.*

Canned chicken or vegetable stocks or broths can save a great deal of time with little sacrifice in flavor when using them in homemade soups. Use low sodium, MSG-free versions whenever possible. I've included recipes for chicken and vegetable broth if you want to take the extra step to make your soup even more delicious and healthy, but prepared broths work well in the following recipes too.

Homemade soups can be easy and economical to make. A batch of black bean soup, for example, can make ten servings for less than the price of a single can of soup. Soup can generally be made in large batches and frozen for convenience. It's worthwhile to learn a few simple methods for making delicious and healthy homemade soups, then use the variations for each recipe to end up with a variety of better-tasting and more nutritious meals.

I have included substitutions and variations that allow you to make good soup even if the exact ingredients specified in the recipe are not in season or are unavailable. For example, if you want to make vegetable soup, you can make it with lentils, barley, and cabbage, or substitute green beans, rice pasta, and fresh spinach. Flexible recipes make it easier to include variety, use seasonal produce, and make quick nutritious meals with what you already have in the pantry. This is especially important for those with picky family members. First, make the soup with vegetables your family likes. Once they learn to enjoy the soup, branch out and try adding new vegetables.

Eating soup for lunch rather than a sandwich or fast food goes a long way toward increasing the amount of vegetables in your diet, as well as decreasing the amount of harmful trans fats, saturated fats, and high glycemic load foods. Even if you're not a cook, you can make homemade soups that you'll like much better than canned soups. You'll be surprised at how easy soups are to make. You'll also be surprised at the difference in taste. Try simple recipes like **Quick Beans and Greens Soup with Ham** or **Vegetable Barley Soup** first. The simplicity of making a meal in one pot is very attractive to busy people. Adding bread or cheese can make your soup a hearty meal. Making a couple varieties of soups per week to serve as a family supper one or two nights a week and to have left over for lunch is an excellent way to eat well and save time and money.

# RECIPES

Ingredients for recipes are listed in order. When instructed to use one ingredient "through" another, then you use that first ingredient, all the ingredients listed between the two, and the final ingredient.

## Quick Beans and Greens Soup with Ham

*This is my favorite quick soup.*

2 teaspoons olive oil
3 carrots, diced
1 large onion, finely chopped
2 cloves garlic, finely minced
7 ounces nitrite-free ham *or* nitrite-free turkey kielbasa, chopped (optional)

4 cups low-sodium chicken or vegetable broth
½ teaspoon black pepper
2 (15-ounce) cans Great Northern beans, drained and rinsed
6 ounces baby spinach

Cook carrots, onion, garlic, and ham in oil 8 minutes, stirring frequently. Add broth and simmer, covered, until carrots are tender, about 15 minutes. Add the beans and pepper. Simmer 3 minutes. Add spinach; remove from heat, stir and serve. 6 servings

*Variation:* Substitute 6 ounces of chopped cabbage for the spinach. Add it at the time you add the broth.

# Kids' Favorite Chicken Noodle Soup

*This simple nutritious soup is popular with kids and has more vegetables than most chicken soups. Freely substitute your favorite vegetables or use fresh or frozen in place of the canned.*

8 cups low-sodium chicken broth
1 bay leaf
5 carrots, sliced
⅓ head of cabbage, shredded
½ pound cubed boneless, skinless
   chicken breast

1 8.5-ounce can no-salt-added
   green peas, drained (about 1 cup)
1 8-ounce can no–salt–added corn,
   drained (about 1 cup)
½ cup diced red bell pepper (optional)
¾ cup alphabet or other small pasta

Boil the broth. Add the carrots, cabbage, and chicken and simmer, covered for 30 minutes. Uncover and add the pasta, corn, peas, and peppers and boil another 5 to 7 minutes until the pasta is done.

*Variation:* You can substitute 1 cup of cooked diced chicken for the chicken breast. Add it with the pasta rather than at the beginning.

# Vegetable Barley Soup

*If you're trying to lose weight, have this soup as an appetizer before lunch and dinner. You'll fill up on a variety of vegetables before other foods tempt you.*

8 cups low-sodium vegetable, beef,
   or chicken broth
5 carrots, sliced
1 large onion, finely chopped
½ small cabbage, shredded
2 cloves garlic, minced

½ cup dried lentils
¼ cup pearled barley
1 14-ounce can tomato sauce
1 teaspoon Italian seasoning
Salt and pepper to taste

Combine all the ingredients from the broth through the barley. Simmer covered for 70 minutes. Add tomato sauce, salt, and pepper. Simmer 10 minutes more and serve.

# Minestrone

*Serve this hearty soup as a meal. Use whatever beans you have on hand or substitute corn or peas. It's especially good served with a grilled cheese sandwich.*

8 cups low-sodium vegetable, beef, or chicken broth
5 carrots, sliced
1 large onion, finely chopped
1 cup uncooked whole-grain pasta
2 cloves garlic, minced
1 (15-ounce) can white beans, drained

1 (15-ounce) can Italian flat beans or other green bean chopped into bite-sized pieces, drained
1 (14-ounce) can tomato sauce
5 ounces chopped spinach leaves
1 teaspoon Italian seasoning
Salt and pepper to taste

Combine all the ingredients from broth through the onion in a large pot. Bring to a boil, then reduce heat. Let simmer, covered, for 30 minutes. Increase heat to medium high. Stir in pasta. Cook uncovered for the amount of time required to cook the pasta according to package directions (10 to15 minutes for most pastas). Reduce heat to medium and add the remaining ingredients. Stir, cover, and simmer 5 minutes until heated through and spinach is wilted.

# Broccoli Soup (dairy-free)

*This healthy soup is nothing more than a vegetable puree thickened with potato rather than butter and cream. It's very light and refreshing. Notice that the following recipes for carrot, spinach, kale, and potato soups are just variations on this simple technique.*

1 medium onion
2 medium red potatoes, peeled and chopped (about ⅔ pound)
2½ cups low-sodium chicken or vegetable broth

1½ pounds broccoli, florets and peeled stalks, chopped
Salt and pepper to taste

Bring broth, potatoes, and onions to a boil. Simmer covered for 10 minutes. Add broccoli and boil 7 more minutes until vegetables are tender. Remove the pot from the heat and puree the soup with an emersion blender or in a blender or food processor until smooth. Season with salt and pepper. Garnish with sour cream or grated cheddar cheese if desired. 4 servings

# Curried Carrot Soup

*The potatoes give this soup a velvety texture.*

1½ pounds of carrots, scrubbed and chopped
1 medium onion, chopped
2 medium red potatoes (about ⅔ pound), peeled and chopped
2 cloves of garlic, minced

2½ cups low-sodium chicken or vegetable broth
2 teaspoons curry powder
1 teaspoon ground ginger
Salt and pepper to taste (optional)

Bring the broth, carrots, potatoes, onion, and garlic to a boil. Simmer covered for 20 minutes or until all vegetables are tender. Add curry powder, ginger, salt, and pepper. Remove the pot from the heat and puree using an emersion blender, or process in batches in a food processor or blender. If soup is too thick, add ½ cup water, milk, or broth. Garnish with fat-free sour cream if desired. 4 servings

# Loaded Potato Soup

2½ pounds of chopped potatoes (peeling is optional)
1 clove of minced garlic
1 medium onion, chopped
2½ cups low-sodium chicken broth

Salt and pepper to taste (optional)
Garnishes: crumbled, cooked bacon; cheddar cheese, chopped scallions, fat-free sour cream

Bring the broth, potatoes, onion, and garlic to a boil. Simmer 15 minutes, stirring occasionally, until potatoes are tender. Remove from heat and puree with an emersion blender or process in batches in a food processor or blender. If soup is too thick, add ½ cup water, milk, or broth. Add salt and pepper to taste. Garnish each bowl of finished soup with ½ strip cooked crumbled nitrite-free bacon, 1 tablespoon grated cheddar cheese, 1 tablespoon chopped scallions, and a dollop of fat-free sour cream. 4 servings

# Spinach Soup

*If you use frozen spinach, a blender or food processor will puree this soup better than an emersion blender. Use the frozen spinach that comes loosely packed in a bag rather than the type that comes frozen in a brick.*

| | |
|---|---|
| 1 pound fresh or frozen spinach | 1 medium onion, chopped |
| ⅔ pound (2 medium) chopped, peeled potatoes | 2½ cups low-sodium chicken broth |
| | ⅛ teaspoon nutmeg (optional) |
| 1 clove of minced garlic | Salt and pepper to taste (optional) |

Boil the potatoes, broth, and onion. Simmer covered until the potato is tender (about 15 minutes). Add the spinach and boil for 2 to 3 minutes more, stirring occasionally. Remove from heat and puree with an emersion blender or process in batches in a food processor or blender. Add nutmeg and the salt and stir. 4 servings

# Kale Soup

*Be sure to remove the tough central stem from fresh kale leaves before chopping. You can also substitute other greens like mustard or turnip greens for the kale or use a combination of greens.*

Substitute 1 pound fresh or frozen kale for the spinach in **Spinach Soup**. Add the kale when you add the potatoes rather than at the end.

# Basic Black Bean Chili

*This ridiculously simple recipe is unbelievably good. Serve over brown rice for a fast and healthy meal you can pull off the shelf on short notice.*

1 (15-ounce can) black beans, drained and rinsed

1 (6-ounce) can tomato sauce *or* 1 (15-ounce) can finely diced tomatoes

2 tablespoons tomato paste *or* ketchup (optional)

1 tablespoon chili powder

1 teaspoon cumin

½ teaspoon garlic powder

Garnishes: grated cheese, fat-free sour cream, chopped cilantro, chopped green onions, avocado slices.

Combine all ingredients in a medium pot over medium heat. Simmer covered for 15 to 30 minutes (or more to give the chili a deeper flavor). Garnish as desired. Serve over brown rice if desired. 4 servings

*Or,* to make chili quick: Combine all ingredients in a microwave safe dish. Microwave on high 3 to 5 minutes, stirring after 2 minutes, until heated through.

*Variations:*

∾ Substitute kidney beans, pinto beans, or other cooked beans for the black beans

∾ Substitute one 15-ounce can of pumpkin puree for the tomato paste and add an additional teaspoon of chili powder for a surprisingly hearty and nutritious chili

∾ Use this bean chili as the filling for burritos: Spoon beans into the center of each tortilla, add cheese if desired. Roll up tortilla and place seam side down on a microwave safe dish. Microwave on high 30 seconds or until hot. Top with salsa or more chili, or the chili garnishes listed above

∾ Add 1 teaspoon curry powder to the chili

∾ Serve with one of the fruit salsas in this book

---

### *Savvy Eating Tip: Meal Planning*

Serve bean, pea, and lentil soups with grains, bread, or cheese to make a meatless meal with complementary (complete) protein.

# Easy Tomato Bean Soup

1 tablespoon olive oil
1 small onion, finely chopped
2 tablespoons finely chopped bell
 pepper *or* 1 jalapeno pepper,
 finely chopped
1 clove finely chopped garlic
2 finely chopped peeled tomatoes *or*
 1 (14.5-ounce) can of chopped
 tomatoes, drained

3 tablespoons tomato paste
1 to 2 teaspoons chili powder
1 teaspoon curry powder
4 cups low-sodium chicken *or*
 vegetable broth
1 (10-ounce) can black, pinto, kidney,
 *or* other type beans, drained
½ cup chopped parsley *or* cilantro
2 to 3 tablespoons cooking sherry

In a large soup pot, heat the oil over medium heat. Add the onions, peppers, and garlic. Cook for 5 minutes, stirring frequently. Add the tomatoes, tomato paste, chili powder, broth, spices, and beans. Simmer 30 minutes, covered. Stir in cilantro or parsley and sherry. 4 servings

# Navy Bean with Bacon Soup

*This hearty soup can be prepared without the bacon, but it adds a great deal of flavor and less than 60 calories and 6 grams of fat to the whole pot of soup. Nitrites are preservatives that have been linked to an increased incidence of cancers. Nitrite-free bacon, sausages, and hams are available at health food stores and some large supermarkets.*

1 cup navy beans
5 cups low-sodium chicken broth,
 vegetable broth, or water
1 large onion, diced
2 carrots, diced
2 cloves garlic, minced

2 slices nitrite-free bacon or a small
 bone from a nitrite-free ham
1 or 2 bay leaves
3 sprigs of parsley, chopped
Salt and pepper to taste

Presoak the beans: In a large pot, cover the beans with water and soak overnight. (Alternatively, cover the beans with water in a large pot. Bring them to a boil for 2 minutes. Remove from heat and let sit, covered, for 2 hours.) Drain the beans and discard the water. Combine the beans with all the remaining ingredients except parsley, salt, and pepper, then simmer covered 1½ hours, stirring occasionally, until beans are tender. Remove the bacon slices and bay leaves and discard. Stir parsley and salt into the soup and serve. (Use 1 teaspoon of salt if using unsalted broth or water. Salt only after tasting if using salted broth.)

# Black Bean Soup

Substitute 1 cup black beans for the navy beans in **Navy Bean with Bacon Soup.** Add 2 teaspoons of chili powder, 1-teaspoon cumin, 1-teaspoon ground coriander, and 1 finely diced bell pepper *or* 1 finely diced jalapeno pepper to the soup pot. Substitute 2 tablespoons chopped cilantro for the parsley. Serve with salsa, fat free sour cream and a splash of cooking sherry.

# Split Pea Soup

1 pound (2½ cups) split peas
6 cups water or chicken or
   vegetable broth
1 bay leaf
2 strips nitrite-free bacon *or* 1 cup
   diced cooked nitrite-free ham

2 onions, diced
2 carrots, sliced
2 cloves garlic, minced
Salt and pepper to taste (about
   1 teaspoon salt if using water or
   unsalted broth)

Pre-soak the peas: In a large pot, cover the peas with water and soak overnight. (Alternatively, cover the peas with water in a large pot. Bring them to a boil for 2 minutes. Remove from heat and let sit, covered for 2 hours.) Drain the peas, and discard the water. Combine all ingredients except salt and pepper in a large soup pot. Bring to a boil, then reduce to a simmer for 45 minutes to one hour or until peas are tender. Remove bay leaf and bacon. Add salt and pepper to taste.

# Lentil Soup

Substitute 1 pound of lentils for the split peas. Omit the pre-soaking step. Add 1 to 2 teaspoons curry powder. Sprinkle with chopped cilantro or parsley and lemon juice if desired. The bacon is optional.

# Tomato Basil Soup

*This flavorful spicy soup is bursting with vitamins and anti-oxidants! Add steamed shrimp, scallops, or white fish at the last minute to make a light elegant meal.*

2 tablespoons olive oil
1 teaspoon crushed red pepper
2 cloves garlic, minced
1 small onion, finely chopped
¼ cup finely shredded carrot
½ cup dry white wine
2 cups roasted red bell pepper, chopped (canned is fine)

3 (14.5-ounce) cans diced tomatoes, drained
½ cup milk (optional)
3 cups loosely packed fresh basil leaves cut into thin ribbons (see technique tip)
½ teaspoon black pepper
½ to 1 teaspoon salt to taste

Heat oil in a large heavy pot over medium heat. Add garlic, crushed red pepper, onion, and carrot. Stir frequently as the vegetables cook for about 3 minutes or until the onion is translucent but not browned. Add wine and increase the heat to high. Continue to cook until the volume of the liquid is reduced by half. Add roasted peppers and tomatoes. Bring to a boil, then reduce the heat, cover, and simmer for an hour. Remove from heat and add the milk and basil while stirring. Puree the soup using a hand-held emersion blender or puree in batches in a blender or food processor. 6 servings

---

### *Savvy Eating Tip: Cutting Technique*

To cut basil into thin ribbons or "chiffonade," stack basil leaves then roll the stack of leaves up into a tight bundle. Using a sharp knife, slice the basil into very thin ribbons.

# Tortilla Soup

*This is a great summertime soup. Ladling the broth over the fresh vegetables at the table makes a great presentation.*

2 ears of fresh corn
1 ripe tomato peeled, chopped and seeded
1 small zucchini diced into ¼ inch pieces
½ red bell pepper diced into ¼ inch pieces
2 medium onions, minced
1 clove of garlic, minced

6 cups of low-sodium chicken or vegetable broth
1 cup diced cooked chicken (optional)
1 teaspoon chili powder
½ teaspoon cumin
Garnishes: shredded cheese, lime wedges, (trans fat-free) tortilla chips, fresh chopped cilantro

Bring broth to a boil. Add onions, garlic, chicken, chili powder, and cumin. Boil about 10 minutes or until the onions are tender. In a separate pot, boil corn 5 minutes, drain, and cut kernels from the cob. Divide corn and other veggies among 5 warm serving bowls. Ladle hot broth over the veggies and garnish as desired. 5 servings

# Curried Pumpkin Soup

*This soup is more complex than most of these recipes, but well worth the effort. If you use all the garnishes, this delicious soup goes from tasty to spectacular.*

2 (15-ounce) cans pumpkin puree
3 tablespoons olive oil
1 large onion, finely chopped
2 carrots, scrubbed and sliced
⅓ cup chopped garlic
½ cup peeled fresh ginger, minced
2 jalapeno peppers seeded and chopped
3 tablespoons curry powder

1 Granny Smith apple, peeled and chopped
1 quart low-sodium chicken or vegetable stock
1 (14-ounce) can unsweetened coconut milk *or* 1 cup fat-free yogurt
2 teaspoons cider vinegar
Zest of one orange, preferably organic

Heat the oil in a large heavy pan over medium heat. Add onions and carrots. Cover and cook, stirring occasionally, for 15 minutes or until vegetables are tender but not brown. Add the garlic, ginger, jalapenos, and curry powder. Cook for 1 minute. Add the pumpkin, apple, and the stock. Bring to a boil then reduce to a simmer. Simmer uncovered for 30 minutes. All vegetables should be soft. Puree the soup with a hand-held emersion blender or puree in batches in a blender or food processor. Add the coconut milk, cider vinegar, salt, pepper, and orange zest. Pour soup in warm bowls and garnish as desired. 8 servings

Possible Garnishes:
- ½ pound medium shrimp, peeled and cooked (2–4 minutes over medium-high heat in 2 tablespoons butter or vegetable oil until just curled and pink)
- ¼ cup chopped cilantro
- ¼ cup dried currants or raisins (pour ¼ cup hot water over them for 5 minutes to plump them up, then drain)
- ½ cup toasted coconut
- 2 tablespoons mango chutney
- ⅓ cup fat-free sour cream *or* yogurt

*Variations:*
- Substitute winter squash for the pumpkin puree: Use 2 pounds of any winter squash peeled and cut into 1-inch cubes, tossed in 2 tablespoons melted butter and roasted at 400 degrees for 30 minutes until tender
- Substitute 2 pounds of cooked, mashed sweet potato for the pumpkin.

# Portuguese Sausage and Kale Soup

2 tablespoons olive oil
3 Yukon gold or red skin potatoes, diced in ½ inch pieces (peeling is optional)
2 medium onions, chopped
6 cloves garlic, chopped
2 bay leaves
1 pound kale, coarsely chopped, stems removed
⅓ to ½ pound nitrite-free (fully cooked) chorizo sausage or turkey kielbasa sausage

1 quart low-sodium chicken or vegetable broth
½ teaspoon salt to taste
½ teaspoon black pepper
1 (15-ounce) can kidney beans, drained and rinsed
1 can diced tomatoes

Heat oil in a large heavy pot on medium high. Add onions and potatoes. Cook and stir for 5 minutes. Add garlic, bay leaves, and kale.

Cover and cook 2 minutes until kale is wilted. Add beans, sausage, and broth and bring to a boil. Reduce heat and simmer covered for 10 minutes until potatoes are tender. Add tomatoes and heat through 3 minutes. 4 servings

*Variation:* substitute peeled, diced sweet potato for some or all of the white potato for added nutrition and flavor.

# Beer and Onion Soup

*Both onions and dark beer contain many antioxidants.*

¼ cup olive oil
4 large onions, thinly sliced
1 teaspoon sugar
1 tablespoon chopped fresh thyme
 (or 1 teaspoon dried)
1 (12-ounce) bottle beer (preferably
 a hearty dark beer)

3 cups low-sodium chicken broth
3 cups low-sodium beef broth
1 teaspoon black pepper
Salt to taste
Garnishes: toasted whole-grain
 croutons, Gruyere or Parmesan
 cheese.

In a large pot, cook oil and onions, stirring occasionally until the onions are softened. Add the sugar and thyme. Cook, stirring often, 15 to 20 minutes until the onions begin to brown and caramelize. Add the beer, scraping up any browned bits in the pan. Add broth and pepper and bring to a boil. Simmer, covered, for 1 hour. Serve over toasted croutons and top with cheese if desired. 12 servings

# Basic Vegetable Broth

*Use this nutritious broth as the base for homemade soups and sauces. Feel free to substitute or add whatever vegetables you have on hand: sweet potatoes, mushrooms, broccoli, potatoes, etc. Adding herbs like thyme, parsley, or bay leaf to add distinctive flavor. Making your own broth rather than using packaged broth is an extra step, but it gives you*

*the opportunity to control the amount of sodium and elim-
inate unwanted additives.*

6 cups water

4 carrots, scrubbed but not peeled

3 stalks celery

1 large onion

⅓ head of cabbage *or* 3 broccoli stalks

2 cloves garlic, unpeeled

1 teaspoon salt to taste

Pepper to taste

Coarsely chop the vegetables so they fit in the pot. Boil covered for 1½ hours.

Place the covered pot in a sink half filled with ice water to cool. Line a colander with two layers of cheese cloth. When the broth is cool enough to handle, pour the broth through a colander into a large container. Place the vegetables in a cheese cloth and squeeze out as much liquid as possible. Discard the vegetables. Strain the broth through cheese cloth if a clear broth is desired. Use the broth immediately or store it in the refrigerator up to 3 days or in the freezer up to 6 months.

# Basic Chicken Broth

*This is the base for many soups and sauces. Making your
own rather than using canned or granulated gives you control over the amount of salt and eliminates additives like
MSG, which may be listed on the label as "natural flavors"
or "flavor enhancer." This homemade broth has better flavor than most purchased types and also contains lots of nutrients from vegetables, which are lacking in many packaged
chicken broths.*

3 pounds chicken, rinsed

1 gallon water

1 teaspoon salt

1 pound coarsely chopped onions

½ pound coarsely chopped celery

½ pound cleaned carrots cut in half

2 cloves garlic, crushed

1 medium sweet potato, quartered

1 bay leaf

4 sprigs parsley

1 sprig fresh thyme

In a very large pot, combine the chicken and water. Boil for 30 minutes while preparing the vegetables. Add the remaining ingredients and boil for another 1½ to 2 hours. Remove the pot from the burner and place the covered pot in a sink full of ice water a few minutes to cool the broth quickly. As soon as it is cool enough to handle, remove the chicken and refrigerate or freeze it for another use. Line a colander with two layers of cheese cloth. Pour the broth though the colander into a large container. Press on the vegetables to squeeze out any broth, then discard the vegetables. Use, freeze, or refrigerate immediately. Broths are very perishable. Fat can easily be skimmed off of the top of the broth after it is refrigerated. Refrigerate up to 3 days or freeze up to 6 months.

# CHAPTER 20

# Eating Your Fruits and Veggies

## *Salads*

It's hard to go wrong when you decide to eat a salad, but the suggestions in this chapter will help you make salads that are so good tasting and so healthy, you'll look forward to eating them every day. For many people, when you say "salad," it conjures up an image of the iceberg lettuce, cherry tomato, and cucumber salad that was made popular by steakhouse chains in the 1970s. If you're one of those people, then read on, because salads were never meant to be that bland and boring. It may be that you like salads a lot more than you think.

A salad should be a combination of the freshest and most nutritious fruits and vegetables available, enhanced but not overpowered by tasty toppings or dressings. While the greens, fruits, and vegetables vary with the seasons, the toppings and dressings vary with your whim.

Keep a variety of salad ingredients on hand so you can enjoy them every day. Prewashed greens will keep in the refrigerator several days. (It's worth buying a salad spinner for quick washing and drying of greens. They really do work.) Chop vegetables and store them separately to keep your salad ingredients fresh longest. You can keep lettuce in your salad spinner, and the other veggies in separate plastic bags or covered bowls. You can often prepare veggies for several days' worth of salads at once, then combine the various ingredients on your plate, salad-bar-style when you're ready for a salad. This works well for families whose members have different tastes. If you plan to bring your salad with you to work or school, it's worth investing in a cooler or lunch box that can keep your salad cold until lunchtime unless you have a refrigerator available.

*You can often prepare veggies for several days' worth of salads at once, then combine the various ingredients on your plate, salad-bar-style when you're ready for a salad.*

*Toss your salad together the night before while you're preparing supper. Keep your dressing in a separate zip-top bag, then your salad is ready to go without hassle or mess in the morning.*

Toss your salad together the night before while you're preparing supper. Keep your dressing in a separate zip-top bag, then your salad is ready to go without hassle or mess in the morning. Create variety by adding different dressings, proteins, and starches to prepared vegetables from your refrigerator. When composing a salad consider the following:

# Tips for Making Great Salads:

~ *Color:* Make your salad as colorful as possible. Use dark green, purple, or red leafy vegetables. Choose red or orange bell peppers, purple onions, purple cabbage, red tomatoes, or bright orange carrots. You feast with the eye first. If you make your salad beautiful to look at, it will be bursting with phytonutrients.

~ *Freshness:* Combine the freshest available ingredients. This means buying (or growing) fresh fruits and vegetables in season. The difference in taste between wax-covered cucumbers shipped from another country in winter and fresh locally grown summer cucumbers is immense. Greens and onions are available year round thanks to growers in California, but they taste best in the spring and fall when they're in season locally. Wait until summer to put fresh ripe tomatoes and cucumbers on your salad and don't bother with them the rest of the year. Make cabbage slaws in the winter and use baby greens, asparagus and artichokes in the spring. Visit the local farmer's market and substitute seasonal vegetables and fruits for old favorites that aren't in season.

~ *Flavor:* A great salad mixes cool, earthy greens and vegetables with *spicy or pungent* ingredients (onions, garlic, peppers, radishes), *tangy* ingredients (vinegar, citrus juices, or mustard), *sweet* ingredients (fresh or dried fruits, honey, sugar, or fruit juices), and *salty* ingredients (salt, capers, olives, or salted nuts). Dressings often provide all four flavors. *Bitter* greens or vegetables can add a fifth dimension.

*Avoid big chunks of anything. If the pieces are so big you can't get more than one or two ingredients in a bite, then it's no longer a salad; it's veggies and dip.*

~ *Texture:* Use a variety of textures to create interest. Mix tender young greens with crunchy nuts or apple chunks. Try delicate leaf lettuces with buttery avocado, black beans, and olives. Pair crisp romaine lettuce with shredded carrots, shredded cabbage,

onion slices, or diced bell pepper. Avoid big chunks of anything. If the pieces are so big you can't get more than one or
two ingredients in a bite, then it's no longer a salad; it's veggies and dip. The pieces should be cut small enough that you
can get several different tastes in one mouthful. However,
unless you're making a slaw, the pieces should be big enough
to provide texture contrast. For a well–rounded, satisfying
salad include as many of the following texture categories as
possible:

- *Crispy:* Crisp lettuce, cabbage, carrot, cucumber, radish, bell
  pepper, summer squash, apple chunks.
- *Starchy:* Whole-grain pasta, boiled potatoes, cooked brown
  rice, quinoa, or barley, whole-grain croutons, baked pita
  crisps, beans, peas.
- *Smooth and creamy:* Avocado, olives, cheese, tofu, boiled
  eggs, dressings.
- *Crunchy:* Sunflower kernels, nuts, whole-grain croutons.

## Making a Salad a Meal

If your salad is to be a complete meal, be sure to include a protein source
with your vegetables. Sliced grilled or baked chicken, lean nitrite-free
ham, boiled eggs, seafood, tofu, beans with corn, beans with pasta, soybeans, cheese, nuts, and seeds are all good choices.

## RECIPES

I've included several specific recipes for salads and dressings. Mix and
match ingredients to make hundreds of different salads that suit your
taste.

*Note:* Recipes for dressings that can be used on a variety of salads are
listed alphabetically at the end of this chapter.

# Mandarin Orange Spinach Salad

*This moist and tangy salad needs no dressing, but a light honey mustard or sesame vinaigrette complements it well.*

Baby spinach leaves, washed
Mandarin orange slices, drained
Purple onion, thinly sliced

Red bell pepper, diced
Toasted sliced almonds

Toss ingredients. Dress if desired with one of the dressing recipes at the end of this chapter.

*Variations:* Substitute roasted, salted sunflower kernels for the almonds. Substitute sliced strawberries, raspberries, diced cantaloupe or melon, apple chunks, peach slices, or mango cubes for the oranges.

# Italian Spinach Salad

*Love onion flavor but hate onion breath? This salad is for you!*

1 medium purple onion, thinly sliced
1 cup roasted red bell peppers,
    diced (fresh or from a jar)
2 teaspoons olive oil

1 (10-ounce) bag baby spinach
    leaves or torn spinach
Pine nuts, toasted
Feta cheese

To caramelize the onions: heat oil in a skillet over medium heat. Add onion. Cover and cook stirring frequently for 10 to 15 minutes until they start to caramelize (brown). Add the peppers and cook another 2 minutes. Cool slightly. Toss with spinach, pine nuts, and feta cheese. Serve with the **Quick Vinaigrette.**

---

### *Savvy Eating Tip: Toasting Nuts*

To toast nuts, place nuts in a baking pan at 350 degrees for 5 minutes, stirring at least once, until lightly browned. Watch them carefully; they burn quickly.

# Green Salad with Caramelized Onions, Bleu Cheese, and Walnuts

Red leaf lettuce
Toasted walnuts
Bleu cheese
Caramelized onion (see recipe for **Italian Spinach Salad** above) or raw, thinly sliced purple onion

Sundried tomatoes packed in oil, chopped
Whole-grain croutons
**Pesto Dressing** *or* **Lemon Olive Oil Dressing**

Combine ingredients in proportions that suit your taste. Toss and enjoy.

# Updated Classic Spinach Salad

1 (10-ounce) bag baby spinach leaves or torn spinach
½ purple onion, thinly sliced
2 boiled eggs chopped
1 cup sliced mushrooms

2 strips nitrite-free bacon, cooked and crumbled
**Honey Mustard Dressing** *or* **Vidalia Onion Dressing**

Toss first 5 ingredients. Serve with dressing. 4 servings

# Greek Salad

1 large head of romaine lettuce
½ medium purple onion, thinly sliced
½ cup feta cheese
1 cucumber, peeled and sliced

Grape or cherry tomatoes, halved
Assorted olives and pepperocini
**Lemon and Olive Oil Dressing**

Thinly slice the lettuce into ribbons (or just tear into bite sized pieces). Toss together salad ingredients and serve with dressing.

# Thai Salad

1 cup chopped cabbage
4 cups mixed salad greens
2 tablespoons chopped onion *or* scallions
½ medium red or yellow bell pepper, diced

2 tablespoons toasted sunflower seeds *or* toasted almonds
¼ cup chopped cilantro

Toss ingredients with **Thai Peanut Butter Dressing** (below). 2–4 servings

# Thai Peanut Butter Dressing

1 tablespoon dark sesame oil
3 tablespoons rice wine vinegar
1 tablespoon soy sauce
1 tablespoon natural peanut butter

½ teaspoon minced fresh ginger (optional)
2 tablespoons water

Whisk together ingredients.

# Favorite Winter Salad

*I keep the ingredients for this salad on hand all winter. It's one of my favorite lunches. I toss in whatever veggies and proteins I have in the refrigerator. Sometimes I substitute chicken for the egg, feta for the cheddar, and add any veggies I can find.*

Baby spinach *or* torn leaf lettuce
Thinly sliced sweet purple onion *or* green onions
Chopped boiled egg
Salted cashews *or* sunflower seeds
Cooked black beans *or* kidney beans, drained and rinsed

Cooked barley, brown rice, *or* whole-grain pasta (optional)
Sharp cheddar cheese, shredded
**Quick Vinaigrette**

Combine ingredients in proportions that suit your taste. Toss and enjoy.

# Favorite Spring Salad

*Dress this salad up for supper with chunks of broiled or roasted salmon or chunk light tuna.*

Mixed baby greens
Leftover new boiled potatoes
Steamed green peas or thawed
   frozen peas
Sliced green onions

Sliced toasted almonds
Shredded carrot
Shredded cheddar or other cheese
Sliced avocado
**Honey Mustard Dressing**

Combine ingredients in proportions that suit your taste. Toss and enjoy.

# Favorite Summer Salad

Romaine or leaf lettuce, torn
Diced ripe red and/or yellow
   tomatoes
Diced cucumber
Thinly sliced sweet onion

Diced red and green bell peppers
Black and/or green olives
Feta cheese *or* mozzarella cheese
Whole-grain croutons (optional)
**Pesto Dressing** or **Quick Vinaigrette**

Combine ingredients in proportions that suit your taste. Toss and enjoy.

*Variation:* Omit the lettuce and croutons. Slice the cucumber, mozzarella cheese, and tomatoes, and arrange them attractively on a platter. Sprinkle them with the remaining ingredients and drizzle with **Pesto Dressing**.

# Summer Tossed Salad

Fresh lettuce of your choice
Diced tomatoes
Diced cucumber
Diced bell pepper
Shredded carrots or summer squash

Sliced green onions
Feta cheese
Steamed shrimp (optional)
**Quick Vinaigrette** or **Roasted Bell
   Pepper Dressing**

Combine ingredients in proportions that suit your taste. Toss and enjoy.

# Favorite Fall Salad

Butterhead or other lettuce, torn
Diced apples or pears
Raisins or dried cranberries
Shredded carrot
Mixed salted nuts *or* toasted pecans

Thinly sliced purple onion
Smoked Gouda cheese
Diced cooked chicken or turkey
  (optional)
**Honey Mustard** or **Quick Vinaigrette**

Combine ingredients in proportions that suit your taste. Toss and enjoy.

# Roasted Vegetable Salad

*Adding sliced roasted or broiled chicken makes this salad
a meal.*

4 cups mixed, chopped (½-inch dice)
  vegetables like tomatoes,
  eggplant, mushrooms, bell
  peppers, onions, and zucchini
2 tablespoons olive oil
¼ teaspoon salt

2 cups cooked quinoa, millet, or
  couscous *or* 4 cups shredded
  romaine lettuce or mixed greens
**Lemon Olive Oil Dressing**
Toasted pinenuts (optional)

Combine chopped vegetables, oil, and salt. Preheat the oven to 450 degrees. Line a baking sheet or roasting pan with aluminum foil, and
spread the vegetables evenly over the foil. Roast for 1 hour, stirring every
20 minutes or until vegetables are tender. Combine ½ of dressing with
the quinoa or lettuce, then top with the vegetables and drizzle with
dressing. Sprinkle with pinenuts. Veggies can be served warm or cold.

# Black Bean and Corn Salad

*This salad stands alone as a side dish or it can be served over salad greens.*

1 tablespoon sugar
2 tablespoons apple cider vinegar or lime juice
1 (15-ounce) can black beans, drained and rinsed
1 cup cooked corn kernels (fresh; frozen, thawed; or no-salt-added canned, drained)

1 jalapeno pepper, seeded and minced
2 scallions, thinly sliced
2 sprigs chopped cilantro
Salt to taste (optional)
Avocado slices (optional)

Combine the vinegar and sugar and whisk well. Add the beans and cilantro and stir to combine. Top with avocado slices if desired. Salt if necessary.

*Variation:* Substitute 2 tablespoons finely diced bell pepper for the jalapeno.

# Marinated Vegetable Salad

*This tasty salad is always popular at potlucks and can be made quickly from cans in your pantry. It tastes best after marinating 8 hours.*

⅓ cup sugar or honey
¾ cup cider vinegar
¼ cup canola oil
½ teaspoon salt
½ teaspoon pepper
1 can no-salt-added peas
1 can French-cut green beans

1 can shoe peg corn
1 can yellow corn
1 small jar of pimientos
1 cup diced celery
1 cup chopped onion
1 cup diced bell pepper

Combine all ingredients from the sugar or honey through pepper. Microwave 1 minute to melt sugar. Whisk well. Drain the canned vegetables and add the remaining ingredients. Stir well. Refrigerate several hours.

*Variations:* Freely substitute different canned, cooked, fresh, or frozen vegetables for the ones specified in the recipe. For an Italian bean salad, substitute a can of kidney beans and a can of white beans for the corn and substitute balsamic vinegar for the cider vinegar. Add a teaspoon of dried Italian herbs.

# Vidalia Onion Dressing

1 large Vidalia or other sweet onion, chopped
1 tablespoon canola oil
½ cup cider vinegar
1 tablespoon honey

1 tablespoon lemon juice
1 teaspoon deli-style mustard
½ teaspoon salt
½ teaspoon pepper
¾ cup canola oil

Heat 1 tablespoon of oil in a large skillet over medium heat. Add onion, cover, and cook, stirring frequently 15 to 20 minutes until the onion is brown and caramelized. Reduce heat if the onion starts to brown too quickly. Process together all ingredients from onions through pepper in a food processor or blender until smooth. While processing, add the remaining oil in a slow steady stream. Makes 1½ cups

# Honey Mustard Vinaigrette

¼ cup honey
¼ cup apple cider vinegar
1 teaspoon salt

⅓ cup walnut *or* canola oil
¼ teaspoon black pepper
2 teaspoons deli-style mustard

Combine ingredients in a jar with a tight fitting lid and shake vigorously.

# Lemon Olive Oil Dressing

¼ cup olive oil
3 tablespoons lemon juice
1 tablespoon red wine vinegar
1 teaspoon Dijon mustard
1 clove finely minced garlic *or* shallot
    *or* ¼ teaspoon garlic powder

¼ teaspoon salt
¼ teaspoon pepper
1 teaspoon honey (optional)

Whisk together all ingredients.

# Sesame Vinaigrette

¼ cup rice wine vinegar (or apple
    cider vinegar)
3 tablespoons honey
2 teaspoons low sodium soy sauce

2 tablespoons toasted sesame seeds
⅓ cup canola oil
1 teaspoon dark sesame oil

Whisk together all ingredients.

# Quick Vinaigrette

1 part balsamic vinegar
2 parts olive oil
Dash of pepper
Dash of Italian or other dried
    herb blend

Dash of garlic powder
Kosher salt or sea salt to taste
    (optional)

Combine vinegar and garlic powder with a whisk or shake in a jar or in a sealable plastic bag. Sprinkle salad greens directly with the desired amount of salt rather than adding salt to the dressing (optional).

*Variation:* For a lighter tasting vinaigrette, substitute white wine vinegar for the balsamic, and walnut oil for the canola.

# Pesto Dressing

1 to 2 cloves garlic
2 cups fresh basil leaves
¼ cup Parmesan cheese

¼ teaspoon salt
⅓ cup white wine vinegar
⅔ cup olive or canola oil

Combine together garlic, basil leaves, Parmesan cheese, and salt in a food processor. Process until finely chopped. Add the vinegar. Pulse. With the processor on, add the oil in a stream through the chute.

# Roasted Bell Pepper Dressing

*This dressing makes a great sauce for shrimp, fish, and chicken too.*

⅔ pound roasted red or yellow bell peppers (about 2 peppers) *or* a 12-ounce jar roasted red peppers, drained
1 clove garlic
¼ cup white wine vinegar

1 teaspoon prepared mustard
½ teaspoon salt
1 teaspoon honey (optional)
¼ teaspoon black pepper
¼ cup olive oil
½ cup chopped fresh basil (optional)

Combine all ingredients from the peppers through the black pepper in a food processor or blender. Process until smooth. Add the oil in a thin stream with processor running. Stir in basil.

# Vinaigrette Slaw

2 tablespoons canola oil
1 tablespoon honey
2 tablespoons cider vinegar
1 tablespoon prepared mustard
1 teaspoon caraway seeds (optional)

½ teaspoon celery seeds (optional)
½ teaspoon salt
1 teaspoon black pepper
1 pound shredded savoy cabbage
2 tablespoons chopped green onions

Combine oil, honey, vinegar, and mustard with a whisk. Combine remaining ingredients. Toss with vinegar mixture and chill.

*Variation*: Substitute packaged coleslaw mix or broccoli slaw mix for savoy cabbage.

# Asian Slaw

¼ cup rice wine vinegar
2 tablespoons low-sodium soy sauce
2 teaspoons dark sesame oil
¼ cup sliced green onions
1 pound finely shredded Napa
  cabbage

2 teaspoons toasted sesame seeds
  (optional)
1 tablespoon chopped fresh cilantro
  (optional)

Combine vinegar, soy sauce, and sesame oil in a large bowl with a whisk. Add remaining ingredients; toss well and chill.

# CHAPTER 21

# Eating Your Fruits and Veggies

## *Fresh Salsas*

Most Americans are familiar with the canned tomato-based salsas available in the chip aisle of the grocery store. Salsa is the number one selling condiment in America. However, many haven't had the pleasure of experiencing fresh salsa. While the canned variety is tasty and nutritious, fresh salsa packs even more vitamins and antioxidants than the heat-processed version and usually has no added salt, sugar, or other unwanted chemicals.

Salsas rarely require any cooking or complicated steps, and usually call for very few ingredients. If you can handle a knife, you can make salsa. Most salsas are a simple mixture of fresh fruits (remember, tomatoes and peppers are technically fruit) and vegetables, especially onions. Salsas are not always spicy and may be sweet. Fresh fruits make salsas vibrant with flavor, so plan to make salsa when quality fresh fruits are available in season.

Salsas are versatile condiments. They can stand alone with chips as a dip, or they make great low-calorie toppings for salads, enchiladas, and meat and fish dishes. Salsas are easy to prepare and have multiple nutritional benefits, but the best reason to try fresh salsa is their incredible taste!

## Fresh Pineapple Salsa

*This salsa is great over grilled chicken or fish.*

1 cup fresh pineapple, cut in ½-inch chunks

⅓ cup purple onion, minced in ¼-inch pieces

1 small jalapeno pepper, minced

2 tablespoons chopped cilantro *or* mint (optional)

Combine pineapple, onion, pepper, and cilantro. Chill if desired. 4 servings

# Mango (or Peach) Salsa

*Try this with southwest chicken. See page 209.*

1 large mango cut in ½-inch chunks *or* 1 cup fresh peaches cut in ½-inch chunks
1 green onion (green and white parts), thinly sliced
2 tablespoons chopped cilantro (optional)

1 small jalapeno pepper, minced (Optional) add 1 to 2 teaspoons of sugar if fresh peaches are not very sweet

Combine fruit, onion, cilantro, and pepper. Chill if desired. 4 servings

# Mixed Fruit Salsa

½ cup fresh pineapple cut in ½-inch chunks
½ cup seeded watermelon cut in ½-inch chunks
½ cup peaches or mango cut in ½-inch chunks
½ cup mild purple onion, minced

1 large jalapeno pepper, minced
½ medium red, yellow or orange bell pepper chopped in ¼-inch pieces
2 tablespoons lime juice (about one lime)
2 tablespoons chopped cilantro (optional)

Combine all ingredients. Chill if desired. 8 servings

# Tomato Salsa

*The size of the tomato chunks is a personal preference. Some like large chunks while others prefer to puree this salsa.*

1 cup peeled, diced, and seeded tomato (one 15-ounce can of diced tomatoes can be substituted)
¼ cup finely chopped onion
1 small jalapeno pepper, seeded and finely chopped

2 tablespoons cilantro, chopped (optional)
¼ teaspoon salt (optional)

Combine all ingredients. Chill if desired. 4 servings

---

### Savvy Eating Tips: Making Salsa

General tips:
- The *size of the chunks* in fruit salsa is important. The chunks need to be small enough to get several different flavors in your mouth at once, but not so small that the fruits lose their character. Onion and pepper pieces should be tiny because their more pungent taste and crunchy texture can overpower the fruit. Therefore, specific sizes are given for the chunks in each recipe; however, adjust the chunk size to your taste.
- *Fresh fruits* are recommended. Canned fruits can be used in off-seasons; however, both taste and nutrition will be sacrificed.
- If fresh fruit is *not very sweet*, consider adding ½ to 1 teaspoon of sugar or honey.

Technical tip:
- *Mincing jalapenos:* Using a cutting board and sharp knife, slice the jalapeno in half, then remove and discard seeds and membranes for these recipes (The seeds and membranes of peppers contain most of the heat of the pepper, while the flesh contains most of the flavor. If you like your salsa fiery hot, you can add the seeds and membranes to the dish.) Chop the jalapeno into ¼-inch strips, then chop the strips into ¼-inch squares. It's wise to wear rubber gloves while chopping hot peppers because the oils from the membranes can irritate your eyes or skin. Wash thoroughly if you don't wear gloves.
- *Have onion or garlic smell on your hands?* Wash hands as usual, then rub your hands on any clean stainless steel spoon. The smell will come off!

## Roasted Tomato Salsa

*Roasting brings out the sweetness in vegetables and intensifies their flavor.*

4 medium peeled tomatoes, quartered
½ cup diced onion
2 small jalapeno peppers, seeded and chopped

1 tablespoon olive oil
2 tablespoons cilantro, chopped (optional)
¼ teaspoon salt (optional)

Toss the tomato halves, onion and peppers with the oil. Line a baking sheet with aluminum foil. Spread the tomatoes, onions, and peppers on the pan and roast them at 400 degrees until tender about (35 to 45 minutes). Place the roasted vegetables, cilantro, and salt into a food processor and pulse several times until desired consistency. (If you prefer a chunky salsa, just mash the mixture by hand rather than in the food processor.)

# CHAPTER 22

# Making Your Veggies More Delicious

When my sister joined an organic farm co-op, she received several large bags full of seasonal produce each week. She got many of the common supermarket variety vegetables like beans, squash, and spinach, but other veggies were more unusual. When she asked the farmer how he would cook the Swiss chard, dikon, patty pan squash, collards, bok choy, or whatever vegetable she found in the bag, he would inevitably say, "I just wilt it in a pan with a little olive oil and garlic."

While most vegetables can be eaten steamed, the farmer was right. There aren't many vegetables that can't benefit from a little garlic and olive oil. You may find you'll come to love some of the vegetables you wouldn't touch as a child when they're prepared using this basic method or one of its variations. It's an invaluable cooking technique because it's simple, flavorful, quick, and healthy.

It's a good idea to chop the garlic first. Studies show that cooking the garlic as soon as it's chopped can decrease some of its nutritive value, so chop it and let it sit there a few minutes. Bottled chopped garlic is fine if you like the taste. Check the label and make sure the only preservative is citric acid (that's vitamin C). About ¼-teaspoon bottled minced garlic or garlic powder can be substituted for each garlic clove if time is short.

While your chopped garlic is sitting on the chopping board becoming more nutritious, prepare the vegetable to be cooked with the garlic. Greens need to be cut or torn into bite-sized pieces. The fibrous central stem should be removed from greens like kale. Green beans and snow peas can be cooked whole. Squash and other solid vegetables should be cut into thin (¼ inch) bite-sized pieces. Some veggies like kale, collards, green beans, bok choy, and broccoli benefit from blanching (boiling them briefly) or steaming them until they're tender-crisp before tossing them in the garlic and oil. Others, like spinach and beet greens, cook so quickly you just throw them in the pan and stir for a couple of minutes. Experiment with other vegetables. Once the basic technique is mastered other sauces can be incorporated.

# Basic Sautéed Spinach with Garlic

*This is the basic method. Feel free to add fresh or dried herbs like thyme, oregano or basil, or black pepper.*

10 ounces washed baby spinach or torn and stemmed large leaf spinach

3 to 4 garlic cloves, minced
3 teaspoons olive oil
⅛ to ¼ teaspoon salt to taste

Heat oil in a large skillet over medium heat. Add the garlic. Stir for 30 seconds. (Skip this step if you're using garlic powder. Just add it with the spinach.) Do not brown. Add the spinach and stir 1 to 2 minutes until spinach is wilted. Season with salt and pepper if desired. 2 to 3 servings

# VARIATIONS:
## Wilted Greens with Garlic, Balsamic Vinegar, and Olive Oil

*If you don't have a steam basket, you can boil the greens in ½ inch of water, then drain.*

1 pound collards, kale, Swiss chard, mustard or turnip greens, chopped bok choy, or shredded cabbage
4 to 5 cloves garlic, minced
1 tablespoon olive oil

1 tablespoon balsamic vinegar (optional)
¼ teaspoon salt to taste

Place a steam basket in a large pot over an inch of boiling water. Place the vegetable in the steam basket, cover, and steam for about 10 minutes until tender-crisp. Remove the steam basket and drain the greens. Pour the water from the pot and turn the heat to medium and add the olive oil. When hot, add the garlic to the pot. Stir for 30 seconds. Do not brown. Add the drained greens and the vinegar and stir for an additional 1 to 2 minutes. Season with salt and pepper to taste.

*Variation:* Skip the steaming step if you would like to use spinach or beet greens.

# Asparagus with Garlic and Olive Oil

*This is a great way to serve asparagus. It's equally good with whole green beans. Just steam them a little longer, about 10 minutes or until tender.*

1 pound thin asparagus
3 cloves garlic, minced

2 teaspoons olive oil
¼ teaspoon salt to taste

Snap tough ends off asparagus spears. Steam the spears for 4 minutes. Pour out water from pan and heat oil in the same pan. Add the garlic and stir for 30 seconds. Do not brown. Add the asparagus and toss to coat.

**Technique Tip:** To mince garlic, using a chef's knife, press down with the palm of your hand on garlic cloves with the broad side of the blade. This will crush the clove and make it easy to peel. Chop off the root end of the clove and discard it and the peel. Finely chop the clove.

# Asian Sauce for Veggies

*This sauce is great on lightly steamed green beans, snow peas, or kale.*

6 cloves garlic, minced
2 teaspoons canola oil
1 tablespoon dark sesame oil
1 teaspoon sugar
3 tablespoons low sodium soy sauce

1½ pounds of desired vegetable (green beans, greens or cabbage, steamed 10 minutes, or raw spinach)

Combine the sesame oil, sugar, and soy sauce in a small bowl. Heat the canola oil in a medium skillet over medium heat. Add the garlic and stir for 30 seconds. Add the sesame oil mixture and the vegetable. Stir over medium heat about 2 minutes until the vegetable is well coated.

# Red Cabbage with Balsamic Vinegar, Mustard, and Raisins

*Substitute collards, kale, or other greens if you like.*

1½ pounds shredded red cabbage
  (or other green leafy vegetable)
6 cloves garlic, minced
3 teaspoons olive oil
1 tablespoon balsamic vinegar

1 tablespoon prepared mustard of
  your choice
¼ cup raisins
1 teaspoon salt
½ teaspoon pepper

Steam the cabbage 10 minutes. Drain. In a separate bowl, whisk together vinegar, mustard, salt, and pepper. Set aside. Heat oil over medium heat. Add the garlic and stir for 30 seconds. Do not brown. Add the cabbage, vinegar mixture, and raisins. Stir over medium heat 3 to 5 minutes to coat.

# Summer Squash with Garlic and Maple Syrup

*This dish will melt in your mouth.*

1 tablespoon olive oil
2 cloves garlic
6 to 7 medium summer squash
  sliced, ¼ inch thick
1 medium onion, diced

¼ teaspoon salt
¼ teaspoon ground black pepper
¼ teaspoon nutmeg (optional)
2 teaspoons pure maple syrup

Heat oil in a large skillet over medium heat. Add all the ingredients from the garlic through the salt. Cook stirring frequently until the squash and onions are tender, about 10 to 15 minutes. Stir in pepper, nutmeg, and syrup and stir another 1 to 2 minutes.

# CHAPTER 23

# Roasting Brings Out the Best

Roasting brings out the best in most vegetables, meats, and some fruits. Roasting vegetables causes the natural sugars they contain to caramelize, making them tender and sweet, and filling your kitchen with a heavenly aroma. Roasting is an extremely easy technique that can be applied to many fruits and vegetables as well as meats and fish at the same time. You can make complete nutritious meals with very little effort. The trick to making perfect roasted vegetables is to cut them into consistently sized pieces so they roast for the same amount of time. Vegetables should be fork tender but not blackened when done.

Roasted vegetables keep two to three days in the refrigerator, so roast a variety of vegetables at the same time. Combine them with pasta, garlic, and olive oil. Toss them in a salad with balsamic vinaigrette. Or serve them with meat or beans and a whole-grain pilaf. Roasted vegetables stand alone as a side dish. They also make great pizza toppings. Roasted vegetables are delicious in many ways, yet easy to prepare.

Rather than giving specific recipes for a few roasted vegetables, I have compiled a chart that enables you to roast whatever vegetables are in season. Pick almost any vegetable, look it up in the chart on page 201, and roast it with olive oil and salt, or one of the seasoning blends listed below.

## Basic Roasted Vegetables

*This is the basic recipe for all roasted vegetables.*

2 cups vegetables                        ¼ to ½ teaspoon salt
1 tablespoon olive oil

Cut vegetables to desired size (see chart on page 201) and toss with oil and salt. Spread vegetables in a thin layer on a cookie sheet or roasting pan lined with aluminum foil and sprayed with cooking spray. Bake at 400 or 450 degrees for specified time (from chart) until vegetables are tender when pierced with a fork. Do not char vegetables.

❧

## Maple-Glazed Roasted Veggies

*This is especially good on winter squash, sweet potatoes, carrots, turnips, and other root vegetables.*

Add 2 teaspoons pure maple syrup for every 2 cups of vegetables and proceed as directed for **Basic Roasted Vegetables.**

# SEASONING BLENDS
## Italian

*This blend is especially good with tomatoes, onions, eggplant, mushrooms, and bell peppers. It's great on pizza, tossed with pasta, or arranged on a platter as an hors d'oeuvre served with thinly sliced crusty bread.*

2 to 4 cups chopped vegetables
1 tablespoon olive oil
¼ to ½ teaspoon salt
2 cloves minced garlic (or 1
   teaspoon garlic powder)

1 tablespoon balsamic vinegar
Fresh or dried basil, thyme, black
   pepper, and oregano to taste
   (Start with ½ teaspoon dried or
   1 to 2 teaspoons of fresh herbs.)

Combine all ingredients. Roast as per chart.

## Southwest

*Sweet potatoes, carrots, winter squash, onions, and potatoes are especially good this way. Try them with roasted chicken or wrapped in a tortilla.*

2 cloves minced garlic *or* 1
   teaspoon garlic powder
½ teaspoon cumin
1 teaspoon chili powder

2 teaspoons brown sugar
1 tablespoon olive oil
¼ to ½ teaspoon salt
2 to 4 cups of chopped vegetables

Combine all ingredients. Roast as per chart on page 201.

# Curried

*Try this with apples, pineapple, sweet potato, carrots, bell peppers, and onions. Serve over brown rice or another whole-grain pilaf. Turmeric, a spice found in most curry powders, can help ward off Alzheimer's disease and auto-immune disorders.*

2 cloves minced garlic (or 1 teaspoon garlic powder)
2 teaspoons curry powder

1 tablespoon olive oil
¼ to ½ teaspoon salt
2 to 4 cups of chopped vegetables

Combine all ingredients. Roast as per chart on page 201.

# Parmesan

*This makes great oven fries with red potatoes or sweet potatoes cut in wedges.*

¼ cup Parmesan cheese
2 teaspoons olive oil
4 cups vegetables

2 tablespoons olive oil
½ teaspoon salt or seasoned salt

Roast vegetables with oil and salt as per chart. Remove them from the oven 15 minutes before they're done, Toss them with an additional 2 tablespoons of oil and cheese and return them to the oven for the remaining 15 minutes.

# Using the Roasting Chart

This chart gives the roasting time needed to roast the listed vegetables, fruits, and meats at *450 or 400 degrees in a single layer* on a roasting pan or baking sheet. If not roasting vegetables in a single layer, you will need *to increase the cooking time* and *stir* the vegetables once or twice while roasting. Vegetables like tomatoes and eggplant that contain a lot of water need to be *stirred* once or twice while roasting anyway to keep them from sticking.

If roasting a combination of vegetables, roast them the length of time required by the vegetable requiring the *longest time*. For example: Tomatoes, eggplant, onions, peppers, and mushrooms in a single layer would take 45 minutes at 450 degrees. In a 1-inch thick layer, the same vegetables would take about an hour at 450 degrees, or an hour and 15 minutes at 400 degrees.

Two different roasting temperatures are given to accommodate cooking meats or breads in the same oven at the same time, making roasted meals easy and time and energy efficient. You can place seasoned chicken breast halves in a bed of diced root vegetables and roast a complete dinner in a single pan in 45 minutes at 400 degrees. If you choose to roast at 450 degrees, you can cook your pizza as you roast vegetables for a salad. Salmon roasts nicely in the same 450-degree oven as your southwestern sweet potatoes or curried carrots, etc.

## Roasted Vegetable Tips

To make clean up quick, line the roasting pan with *aluminum foil* and spray the foil with cooking spray.

If you're roasting a variety of vegetables that require different lengths of time, place each type of vegetable on a *separate* piece of foil to make it easy to remove one set of vegetables if it gets done earlier than the rest.

You can chop the vegetables and toss them with oil several hours *in advance* and keep them in a covered container *in the refrigerator* until you're ready to roast them. Drain them before placing them on the roasting pan.

Always *preheat* the oven before roasting.

## Roasting Chart

| Item to be roasted | Time in minutes at 450 degrees | Time in minutes at 400 degrees | Size of pieces | Comments |
|---|---|---|---|---|
| Apples | 20 | 25 | ½-inch chunks | |
| Asparagus | 20 to 25<br>30 | 25 to 30<br>35 | Pencil-thin spears<br>Thick spears | |
| Beets | 40 | 45 | ½-inch cubes | No need to peel beets if you scrub them well. Cook fresh beet tops as as you would spinach. |
| Broccoli | 20 to 25 | 25 to 30 | Florets | |
| Brussels sprouts | 25 | 30 | Cut larger ones in half, small ones whole | |
| Carrots | 30<br>40 | 35<br>45 | ½-inch chunks<br>"baby carrots" | Cut large carrots in half before cutting into specified lengths |
| Eggplant | 35<br>35 to 45 | 45<br>45 to 60 | 1-inch cubes<br>½-inch thick wheels | Stir or turn slices over once or twice during cooking time. Cook with peppers, onions, tomatoes, and mushrooms. You can start the eggplant 20 minutes before the other veggies if you like. |
| Green beans | 20 | 25 | Whole | |
| Mushrooms | 30<br>25<br>20 | 35<br>30<br>25 | Portabello caps<br>Button, whole<br>Button, ¼-inch slices | Add a splash of balsamic vinegar to basic roasted mushrooms |
| Onions | 20 to 25<br>30 | 25<br>35 | Diced<br>¼-inch rings | |
| Parsnips | 35 | 45 | ½-inch chunks | Cut large end in half before cutting into chunks |

| Item to be roasted | Time in minutes at 450 degrees | Time in minutes at 400 degrees | Size of pieces | Comments |
|---|---|---|---|---|
| Pears | 25 | 35 | Halves | Cut in half and scoop out core with a spoon. Drizzle with 1 teaspoon honey and 1 tablespoon sherry or white wine. |
| Peppers | 15 to 20 | 20 to 30 | Jalapeno, halved and seeded | Cooking time depends on thickness of the pepper's flesh. Flesh should be soft when done. It is OK to char the skin of halved peppers if you plan to remove the skin. Skin is removed most easily if it's blackened, then cooled in a paper bag. Diced peppers do best when combined with diced onions while cooking. |
|  | 20 to 30 | 30 to 40 | Bell or ancho, halved and seeded |  |
|  | 15 to 25 | 25 to 35 | Any type, diced |  |
| Pineapple (fresh) | 25 | 30 | 1-inch cubes | A little sugar, maple syrup, or honey tastes great along with a small amount of salt and oil. |
|  | 20 | 25 | ½-inch rings |  |
| Potatoes | 35 | 45 to 60 | ⅛ potato lengthwise wedges | Leave skins on for better nutrition. |
|  | 30 | 35 | ½-inch cubes |  |
|  | 60 |  | whole (medium) |  |
| Squash (summer) | 30 to 35 | 35 to 40 | ½-inch wheels | Stir during cooking. Tastes best when cooked with peppers and onions. |
|  | 20 to 25 | 25 to 30 | Very thinly sliced (OK to let the pieces overlap.) |  |
| Squash (winter) | 45 | 60 | ½ seeded acorn, butternut, or other medium sized winter squash | Try substituting 1 teaspoon butter or trans-fat-free margarine and 2 teaspoons brown sugar or maple syrup per squash half for the oil and salt. |
|  | 30 | 35 to 40 | 1-inch cubed, peeled |  |

| Item to be roasted | Time in minutes at 450 degrees | Time in minutes at 400 degrees | Size of pieces | Comments |
|---|---|---|---|---|
| Sweet potatoes | 35 | 45 | ⅛ potato wedges | |
| | 30 | 35 | ½-inch cubes | |
| | 60 | 60 to 75 | whole, skin on | |
| Tomatoes | 30 | 40 | Medium, halved | |
| | 25 | 30 | Cherry, halved or 1-inch cubed | |
| Turnips | 35 | 45 | ¼ small turnip | Pick young tender turnips. They're great with maple syrup. |
| | 30 | 35 | ½-inch cubes | |
| Chicken | | 60–70 | 2½ to 3 pound whole (not stuffed) | Cooking times are approximate and vary considerably depending on the size of the piece of chicken. Internal meat temperature should reach 180 degrees. Juices should be clear, and the interior of the meat should no longer be pink. |
| | 35 | 40 | Boneless skinless breasts | |
| | | 45–60 | White pieces, bone in | |
| | | 50–60 | Dark pieces, bone in | |
| Fish | 10 to 12 minutes per inch of thickness | | Fillets, fresh or thawed | The fish will flake easily when a fork is inserted into the fillet and turned. |
| | 15 to 20 | | Frozen fillets ½-inch thick | Season with salt and pepper. Drizzle white fish with olive oil, salt, and lemon juice if desired. |
| | 10 to 15 | | Frozen fillets ¼-inch thick | |

# CHAPTER 24

# Shortcuts to Poultry and Fish

## Poultry and Fish the Easy Way

Make the preparation of healthy meats like poultry and fish as simple and safe as possible. Because humanely raised poultry and wild fish tend to be expensive, buy them in large quantity whenever they're on sale and freeze what you don't plan to use right away. Boneless skinless chicken breasts, fish fillets, and seasoned, cooked ground chicken are especially handy to have on hand in the freezer because they can go from the freezer to the table in 20 minutes.

Raw poultry can be dangerous stuff. You can't tell if the chicken you just bought is contaminated with salmonella, so you always need to treat it like it is contaminated. This means thoroughly cleaning your hands and utensils with warm soapy water, and cleaning counter tops, sinks (including faucet handles), and cutting boards with a 1:20 Clorox solution immediately after handling poultry, eggs, raw meat, or fish. Don't use the same utensils or cutting boards for raw meat and vegetables.

Because dealing with raw meat can be a chore, it's wise to deal with it only once or twice a week. This can be accomplished by preparing large quantities of poultry at once and freezing it in convenient one meal-sized packages for later use. Two types of poultry are particularly practical for buying in bulk and freezing: boneless skinless chicken breasts and lean ground turkey or chicken, so I'll focus on them.

On your meat preparation day, you can prepare one or more marinades for your meat and freeze your chicken in the marinade so there is no mess or extra preparation steps on the day you cook them. Boneless skinless breasts can also be frozen plain and seasoned the day you cook them.

Ground turkey and chicken have so many uses. It's great to be able to pull a package of seasoned, cooked ground turkey or homemade turkey sausage out of the freezer, just briefly thaw it in the microwave and add it to sauces, chili, pasta dishes, and casseroles.

The reasons are twofold:

1. Avoiding unwanted ingredients like excessive sodium and MSG
2. Cost

Buying fresh poultry is much cheaper than prepared items. Use your store of frozen poultry to add to the many pasta, rice, and vegetable dishes in this book that list a variation that calls for cooked chicken, poultry sausage, or cooked ground poultry.

Frozen chicken breasts or fish fillets can provide a quick healthy protein while you concentrate your efforts on preparing delicious vegetable and whole-grain dishes. The following methods of advanced preparation and freezing save money, time, and effort.

# Boneless Skinless Chicken Breasts

### FREEZING

Separate the individual breasts and place them on a baking sheet lined with aluminum foil. Place them in the freezer for 30 minutes (this keeps them from sticking to each other when they are frozen) then transfer them to freezer bags. Place the number that you would usually cook for your family in each bag. Press any air out of the bags before sealing. Label each bag with contents and the date. Freeze up to 6 months.

### MARINADES

You can freeze chicken breasts with just about any seasoning or marinade. Mix your marinade (see recipes below) in a medium or large bowl. Add the breasts and stir to coat. Place the breasts in freezer bags. Divide any excess marinade among the bags then seal. Once the bags are sealed, lay them flat on the counter and pat them flat so that the individual breasts are not overlapping, and release any air bubbles. Wipe the outsides of the bags clean with a paper towel dipped in 1:10 Clorox solution. Label and freeze for up to 6 months.

### THAWING

Thaw poultry in its bag in the refrigerator overnight or thaw in the microwave: Place the bag of plain or marinated chicken on a microwave safe dish. Open the bag and microwave on defrost for 3 minutes. Rotate and separate the breasts as much as possible. Microwave on defrost another 2 to 3 minutes (depending on the size of the package) until the breasts are almost thawed. Proceed with recipe.

### ROASTING

Place fresh or semi-thawed breasts in a roasting pan lined with foil. Season as desired. Add vegetables prepared for roasting if desired (see chapter 23 on roasting vegetables). Place the breasts on the pan so that they're not touching. Roast at 450 degrees for 35 minutes or at 400 degrees for 45 minutes or until juices run clear. Roasting time varies considerably depending on the size of the breasts.

### BROILING

Position oven rack 4 to 6 inches from the heat source. Preheat broiler. Line a roasting pan with aluminum foil. Place the fresh or nearly thawed boneless skinless chicken breasts on the aluminum. Season as desired. If the breasts have been marinated, let excess marinade drip off before placing the breast on the pan. (Marinade on the pan will burn before the chicken is done.) Broil 7 to 8 minutes on each side. The size and thickness of the chicken breast will determine the exact broiling time. Partly frozen pieces will need an extra minute or two on each side. Juices should run clear and no pink should be visible when you cut into the center of the breast.

### LEFTOVERS

Leftover cooked meat that you don't plan to eat within the next 2 days can be chopped into bite-sized pieces, placed in freezer bags, labeled, and frozen for up to 3 months. The frozen cubed meat can be added directly to most soups and casseroles that require cooking. It also thaws quickly in the refrigerator or microwave.

## Crock-pot Chicken

Whole chicken, chicken parts, chicken breasts, and boneless skinless breasts can be placed in the crock-pot with water and vegetables in the morning before work, set on "low," and left until suppertime. (Follow the instructions included with your crock-pot.) When you come home, your home will be filled with a delicious aroma, and you'll have not only cooked chicken, but broth and veggies too.

If you're rushed in the morning, prepare the ingredients for the crock-pot the night before while you're preparing supper. Place the veggies and chicken in the ceramic pot the night before, cover, and *put the ceramic pot in the refrigerator overnight.* In the morning, place the ceramic pot into the crock-pot heating unit, add the water, and turn it on. No chopping smelly onions or handling raw chicken first thing in the morning. What's more, because you prepared the ingredients the night before, you clean up only once for two meals. Strain and save the broth for other soups and recipes. (If you do not plan to use it within 24 hours, freeze it.) Any leftover chicken that won't be used within two days can be frozen as described in the "leftovers" section.

Use your favorite crock-pot recipe or just place marinated chicken breasts from one of the recipes below on a bed of chopped onions in the pot. Add enough water to make it 2 inches deep and set on low in the morning to have chicken ready for supper.

# Seasoned Ground Poultry

*This recipe easily doubles and triples if you want to prepare a large amount for freezing.*

| | |
|---|---|
| 1 onion, finely chopped | 2 teaspoons olive oil |
| 2 cloves of garlic, minced | ¼ teaspoon salt |
| 1 pound of ground chicken or turkey | |

In a large skillet, heat the oil over medium heat. Add the onions and garlic. Cook, stirring occasionally, 5 minutes, until soft. Add the ground poultry. Break up the poultry into small bits with a spatula while cooking, stirring often until no pink remains. At this point the poultry is ready to add to pastas, sauces, pilafs, chilis, and other dishes, or freeze as below.

*Variation:* For chicken or turkey " sausage," add 1 cup minced fresh basil, 1 teaspoon crushed fennel seeds, and 1 teaspoon crushed red pepper as you cook the poultry. Use in pasta dishes or on pizzas.

### Freezing

Allow the mixture to cool slightly and place the desired amount into freezer bags. Pat the bags flat and press out any excess air. Label and date the bags, and freeze up to 6 months.

# Marinades and Seasonings

*Because uncooked fish or poultry can contaminate the marinade, the remaining marinade should be thrown out, unless you boil it for at least 6 minutes. Fish should be marinated just before cooking. It doesn't freeze well marinated.*

## Southwest Marinade

1 tablespoon brown sugar
4 teaspoons chili powder
1 teaspoon cumin
½ teaspoon salt
2 teaspoons lime, lemon, *or* orange
  zest (preferably from organic fruit)
  (optional)

¼ cup lime, lemon, orange, *or*
  pineapple juice
1½ to 2 pounds chicken or fish

Whisk together sugar and lime juice. Marinate fresh fish for 15 minutes and chicken for 30 minutes *in the refrigerator* before roasting or broiling.

Variation: Dry rub. Omit the juice. Rub the dry ingredients on the fish or chicken, drizzle each piece with a teaspoon of olive oil, and broil or roast. This is my favorite seasoning for roasted salmon.

## Asian Marinade

2 tablespoons soy sauce
1 tablespoon dark sesame oil
1 teaspoon sugar

6 cloves of garlic, minced
1 to 1½ pounds of chicken, fish,
  or tofu

Combine all ingredients. Marinate fish for 15 minutes and chicken and tofu for 30 minutes before roasting or broiling. (Cut tofu into chunks and cook tofu and marinade in a skillet over medium-high heat 7 to 10 minutes, turning at least once, until the tofu is heated through and the marinade is thickened.)

## Italian Marinade

¼ cup olive oil
¼ cup balsamic *or* red wine vinegar
½ teaspoon salt
2 cloves minced garlic *or* 1 teaspoon garlic powder

1 teaspoon dried Italian herbs (any combination of thyme, oregano, basil, etc.)
¼ teaspoon black pepper
2 pounds of chicken or fish

Combine all ingredients. Marinate fish 15 minutes and chicken 30 minutes in the refrigerator, then broil or roast.

## Herb Marinade

¼ cup olive oil
¼ cup lemon juice
2 teaspoons white wine or white wine vinegar
2 tablespoons mixed dried herbs *or* ½ cup mixed chopped fresh herbs (parsley, thyme, rosemary, oregano, marjoram, basil, chervil, etc.)

½ teaspoon salt
1 teaspoon black pepper
2 pounds chicken or fish

Combine all ingredients. Marinate fish up to 15 minutes and chicken for 30 minutes, then roast or broil.

## Buffalo-Style Hot Chicken

*If you like Buffalo-style chicken wings, this one is for you. You can use wings if you like, but using boneless, skinless chicken breasts cut into strips eliminates a lot of saturated fat.*

2 tablespoons olive or canola oil
1 tablespoon Tobasco or other hot sauce
¼ to ½ teaspoon salt

1 pound chicken breasts cut into strips *or* 1 pound of chicken wings
½ cup flour

Sprinkle chicken with salt. Roll the chicken in the flour to coat. Combine the oil and Tobasco sauce. Coat the chicken in the sauce. Preheat broiler. Place the chicken on a foil-lined baking sheet. Broil 6 inches from the heat for 5 to 7 minutes on each side until done. Juices should run clear, and there should be no trace of pink.

# Easy Rules of Thumb for Cooking Fish Fillets

### BROILING

Place fresh fillets on an aluminum foil-lined baking sheet. Use a marinade or just sprinkle with salt and pepper or other seasonings. White fish benefit from drizzling with a small amount of olive oil. Oily fish like salmon don't need added oil. Broil 4 to 6 inches below the heat source, 5 to 6 minutes for every ½ inch of thickness. When done, fish should flake easily when a fork is inserted and twisted.

### ROASTING

Place fresh or thawed fillets on an aluminum foil-lined baking sheet. Season as desired. Bake in a 450-degree oven for 5 to 6 minutes per ½ inch of thickness. When done, fish should flake easily when a fork is inserted and twisted.

Thin frozen fillets can be cooked without thawing. Roast ¼ inch-thick fillets for 10 minutes, and ½ inch-thick fillets for 15 minutes, until they test done.

# CHAPTER 25

# Egg Dishes

Eggs are a healthy protein option if eaten in moderation. They're also cheap, versatile, and easy to prepare on a moment's notice. Limiting your whole egg consumption to seven a week is probably a good idea for most of us, but you don't need to limit your consumption of eggs if you just use the whites. Egg whites are an excellent source of protein. You can substitute two egg whites for one whole egg in most recipes.

Vegetable and egg combinations are a great way to start your day off with satisfying protein and healthy veggies. You can also throw together a quick and nutritious supper in a hurry. The egg scrambles can be made with tofu in place of the eggs if you wish. Just substitute one ounce of crumbled firm or extra firm tofu for each egg and heat through for eight to ten minutes.

## Curried Veggie Scramble

*This scramble is full of vibrant color and antioxidants from the carrots, parsley, onions, and spices. What a powerful way to start your day.*

5 eggs, beaten *or* 5 ounces firm
  tofu, crumbled
½ small purple onion *or* 3 scallions,
  finely chopped
1 large carrot, finely shredded

2 teaspoons olive oil
4 to 5 sprigs of parsley, chopped
2 teaspoons curry powder
Salt and pepper to taste

Heat the oil in a medium skillet. Add the onions, carrots, and curry powder. Cook, stirring often, for 8 minutes, until the vegetables are tender. Add the eggs (or add the tofu and just heat through). Do not stir until the eggs appear almost set, but not brown on the bottom. Stir the egg mixture until the eggs are just firm. Remove from heat. Sprinkle with parsley, salt, and pepper. 2 servings

# Mexican Style Scramble

*This spicy dish is great for breakfast with whole-grain tortillas, or serve it with a salad for supper.*

8 eggs, beaten
¼ cup skim milk
2 teaspoons olive oil
1 large onion, finely chopped
1 red or green bell pepper, finely diced
1 small jalapeno pepper, seeded, and minced, *or* 1 (4.5-ounce) can chopped green chilies, drained

1 medium tomato, diced *or*
    1 (14.5-ounce) can diced tomatoes, well drained
1 teaspoon chili powder
Cooking spray
1 cup grated sharp cheddar cheese (optional)
Salt and pepper to taste

In a medium skillet, heat oil over medium heat. Add the onions and bell peppers, stirring frequently, for 5 minutes, until they're tender. Add the jalapenos (or chilies), tomatoes, and chili powder. Cook stirring occasionally for 5 minutes. Drain off any excess liquid and put the pepper mixture in a bowl and keep warm. Wipe the skillet with a paper towel and return it to medium heat. In a medium bowl, whisk together the eggs and milk. Spray the skillet with cooking spray and add the egg mixture. Do not stir until the eggs appear almost set but not brown on the bottom, then stir the eggs until they are set. Stir in the pepper mixture and remove from heat. Season with salt and pepper and sprinkle with cheese if desired. 4 servings

# Garden Scramble

8 eggs
¼ cup skim milk
2 teaspoons olive oil
1 large onion, finely chopped
1 clove of garlic, minced
1 cup button (or other) mushrooms, sliced
1 red bell pepper, diced

1 small unpealed zucchini, finely diced
Cooking spray
Salt and pepper to taste
1 green onion thinly sliced
¼ cup grated Parmesan cheese (optional)

Heat the oil in a medium skillet over medium heat. Add all the ingredients from the onion through the zucchini. Cook, stirring frequently, for

8 minutes or until the vegetables are tender. Drain any excess liquid from the mixture and place the veggies in a bowl and keep them warm. Wipe the skillet with a paper towel and return it to medium heat. Whisk together the eggs and milk in a medium bowl. Spray the skillet with cooking spray and add the egg mixture. Do not stir until the mixture just starts to set on the bottom. Then stir until the eggs are set. Add the veggies and remove from heat. Season with salt and pepper and sprinkle with green onion and cheese if desired. 4 servings

# Crustless Spinach and Feta Quiche

2 teaspoons olive oil
1 small onion, finely diced
1 clove of garlic, minced
7 ounces fresh spinach, torn
Cooking spray
4 eggs

1 cup skim milk
4 ounces feta cheese, crumbled
¼ teaspoon nutmeg (optional)
¼ teaspoon salt
¼ teaspoon pepper

In a medium skillet, heat the oil over medium heat. Add the onions and garlic. Cook stirring occasionally for 5 minutes. Add the spinach and stir for 2 to 3 minutes, until the spinach is wilted. Remove from heat and cool slightly.

Spray a 2-quart casserole with cooking spray. Whisk together the eggs, salt, pepper, nutmeg, and milk. Combine the egg and spinach mixtures and bake at 350 for 1 hour until set. 4 servings

*Variation:* Top quiche with thin tomato slices in a decorative pattern before baking.

# CHAPTER 26

# Beans: The Super Food

The humble bean is one of nature's super foods. Beans are versatile, inexpensive, high in protein, high in fiber, and full of nutrients like folate. They're also filling and satisfying. Beans are a food we would benefit from eating every day. To help prevent heart disease, fight cancer, ward off diabetes, and control your appetite, aim for eating at least a half cup a day or four cups per week.

Eating beans in place of meat several times a week can go a long way toward decreasing your saturated fat intake and increasing the amount of vegetables and fiber in your diet. It can also save you a lot of money.

Try bean side dishes like **Carolina Caviar** to round out a meal, or make beans the main dish with bean burritos or red beans and rice. Have a nutritious meal but feel like you've had a mini-party when you have hummus or black bean dip with pita chips for lunch. Be careful though, once you've tried these homemade dips, you may never settle for dip from a jar again. The recipes for bean soups and chilies found in the soup section of this book make hearty lunches and satisfying suppers. Even if you're not a bean fan now, try some of the recipes in this book. You may change your mind. Learn to love beans: they're good for your heart.

## Best Black Beans and Rice

*This is a favorite of my whole family.*

1 tablespoon olive oil
1 large onion, finely diced
1 teaspoon garlic powder
2 teaspoons curry powder
1 teaspoon low-sodium soy sauce
　or Bragg's Liquid Aminos

2 (15-ounce) cans black beans,
　drained
1 cup brown rice or quinoa
　prepared according to package
　directions

Heat oil in a medium pot over medium heat. Add onion, cover, and cook, stirring occasionally, for 8 to 10 minutes, until onion is translucent and tender. Add garlic powder, curry powder, and soy sauce. Cook, uncovered, stirring occasionally, for 2 minutes. Add beans and heat through. Serve over rice.

# Carolina Caviar

*This makes a great side dish. You can also serve it with whole-grain crackers or pita chips for an hors d'oeuvre or a snack.*

2 (15-ounce) cans black-eyed peas, drained and rinsed
1 small sweet purple onion, finely diced
1 small red or green bell pepper, finely diced

¾ cup coarsely chopped pimento or jalapeno-stuffed green olives
2 tablespoons cider vinegar
2 teaspoons sugar
1 tablespoon canola oil

Combine all ingredients. Chill.

# Red Beans and Rice

*This is a southern staple for good reason. It's tasty, healthy, satisfying, cheap, and easy to make.*

2 teaspoons olive oil
1 large onion, diced
1 green pepper, diced
4 cloves of garlic, minced
¼ teaspoon cayenne pepper
½ teaspoon black pepper
1 bay leaf

2 (15-ounce) cans dark red kidney beans, drained
1 cup brown rice
2 cups low-sodium chicken broth *or* 2 cups water plus ½ teaspoon salt
Hot sauce to taste

Heat the oil in a large pot over medium heat. Add the onions, green peppers, garlic, pepper, and bay leaf. Cook, stirring frequently for 5 minutes. Add the beans, rice, and broth. Cover and bring to a boil, then reduce heat, and simmer for 1 hour, until rice is done. Remove the bay leaf. Fluff rice with a fork and let stand, covered, for 10 minutes. Add hot sauce to taste.

# Hoppin' John

Substitute black-eyed peas for the red beans in **Red Beans and Rice**. Add 1 cup cooked corn after the beans and rice are done (optional).

# Hummus

*Tahini is a paste made from sesame seeds that gives this classic Middle Eastern dip its characteristic flavor. If you don't have tahini, you can make the dip without it.*

1 clove garlic
1 (19-ounce) can chickpeas, drained
  (about 2 cups)
2 tablespoons lemon juice

1 tablespoon low-sodium soy sauce
1 tablespoon tahini
2 tablespoons parsley

Process all ingredients in a food processor until smooth. Serve with whole-grain pita.

# Black Bean Dip

*The darker the bean, the more antioxidants it contains. Black beans rank number one in antioxidants.*

2 teaspoons olive oil
1 small onion, finely chopped
2 cloves garlic, minced
2 teaspoons chili powder
1 teaspoon cumin

1 (15-ounce) can black beans,
  drained
2 tablespoons tomato paste
Salt to taste
Chopped cilantro (optional)

Heat olive oil in a medium-sized skillet over medium heat. Add the onion. Cook, stirring frequently, for 8 minutes, until onions are tender. Stir in the garlic, salt, and spices, and stir over medium heat 2 minutes. Remove from heat and let cool slightly. Combine the tomato paste, beans, and onion mixture in the bowl of a food processor. Process until desired consistency. (If you prefer a chunky dip, just mash beans with other ingredients in a bowl.) Sprinkle with chopped cilantro. Serve with pita or tortilla chips.

*Variation:* This bean dip makes awesome burritos. Just substitute the dip for the refried beans and follow the assembly and heating directions below.

# Quick Refried Bean Burritos

1 can fat-free refried beans
4 whole-grain large tortillas
  (made without trans fat)
2 green onions, chopped

4 ounces shredded Monterey
  Jack cheese
1 cup prepared salsa (store-bought
  or one of the recipes in this book)

Spoon ¼ of the beans on to each of the tortillas. Sprinkle them with cheese and onion. Roll the tortillas around the bean mixture and place seam-side down in a 9-inch square baking dish. Pour the salsa over the tortillas, making sure that the salsa covers all of the tortillas. Bake at 350 degrees for 35 minutes or until bubbly.

*Variation:* Rather than baking the prepared burritos, microwave them for 1 to 2 minutes on high or until hot.

# White Beans With Pesto and Spinach

2 teaspoons olive oil
4 cloves garlic, minced
10 ounces fresh spinach, torn
1 (15-ounce) can white beans,
  drained
½ cup homemade or commercial
  basil pesto

¼ cup grated Parmesan cheese
¼ cup pine nuts *or* walnut pieces,
  toasted 5 minutes at 350 degrees
2 cups cooked brown rice *or*
  whole-grain pasta, *or* toasted
  whole-grain bread, broken into
  bite-sized pieces.

Heat the oil in a medium-sized skillet over medium heat. Add the garlic and stir and cook 30 seconds. Add the spinach and beans and stir 3 minutes or until the spinach is wilted. Remove from heat and stir in pesto. Serve over brown rice, pasta, or toast. Sprinkle with cheese and pine nuts.

# CHAPTER 27

# Great Grains

## Whole-Grain Pastas, Pilafs, and Cereals

With the growing popularity of the low-carb diet, many of our favorite comfort foods and staples are being avoided by dieting Americans. While there's no faster way to put on the pounds than to frequently indulge in *refined* carbohydrates, whole-grain pilafs, pastas, and cereals are key to preventing cancer, regulating the colon, and optimizing our cholesterol profiles to help prevent heart attacks and strokes. They're an integral part of a disease-prevention diet as well as a diet that helps you loose weight and keep the weight off.

However, you can eat too much of a good thing. Americans tend to eat too many carbohydrates and too few vegetables, our other disease-fighting allies. An easy way to remedy this situation is to increase the ratio of vegetables to grains in pasta and grain dishes. The dish ends up being pleasing to the eye and palate, while satisfying you with fewer calories and more nutrition.

It's important to use whole-grain pastas. A good variety of shapes and types of whole wheat, brown rice, and other whole-grain pastas are now available in most supermarkets.

Whole grains like brown rice take longer to cook than the refined varieties, but you can cook two or three day's worth at once and reheat them in the microwave when needed. There are also quick cooking varieties of brown rice and barley that are ready in around twenty minutes. Recipes are given for a specific grain, but other whole grains like barley or quinoa can be substituted.

Breakfast is a great time to eat whole grains. The key to satisfaction is adding proteins like milk, yogurt, nuts, or soy to cereals. They make a hearty meal that lasts all morning. Try the **Fruit and Nut Breakfast Pilaf** and the **Power-Packed Morning Oats** recipes in this chapter as well as the healthy pancake recipes in the bread chapter. You'll feel so satisfied you won't be tempted by the vending machine at work anymore!

Pasta, rice, and cereals are great energy foods, which means they contain a lot of carbohydrate calories. Grains can be a part of a healthy diet if you eat them in moderation, choose them wisely, and choose what accompanies them wisely as well.

# RECIPES

## Easy Pasta and Veggies with Tomato Sauce

*This is a great way to sneak in a few veggies for picky eaters. You may need to use fewer veggies at first if you're feeding extremely veggie phobic eaters.*

| | |
|---|---|
| 1 pound box of whole-wheat pasta | 1 (15-ounce) can tomato sauce |
| 2 carrots, grated | (preferably low-sodium) |
| 2 broccoli stalks, peeled and grated | Grated cheese (optional) |

Bring 8 cups water with ½ teaspoon salt to a boil. Add the carrots, broccoli, and pasta. Cook as directed on the pasta box. Serve with hot tomato sauce and cheese if desired. 4 to 6 servings.

*Variations:*
- ∾ Substitute 1 cup finely grated cabbage for the broccoli
- ∾ *Pasta with meat sauce:* Add ½ pound ground chicken or turkey cooked with 1 diced onion and 2 cloves of minced garlic to the sauce.
- ∾ *Baked Pasta with cheese:* Combine the pasta and sauce in a casserole dish and top the dish with 2 cups fat-free cottage cheese mixed with 1 teaspoon Italian herbs, and 1 cup grated pizza cheese. Bake at 350 degrees for 30 minutes until bubbly.

## Pesto and Veggies

*The beauty of this simple tasty dish is that you make everything in one pot This is my children's favorite pasta dish.*

| | |
|---|---|
| ½ teaspoon salt | ½ to ¾ cup homemade or prepared |
| 2 carrots, sliced into wheels | basil pesto (to taste) |
| 1 pound box of whole-grain pasta | ¼ cup Parmesan or feta cheese |
| 2 cups broccoli florets | (optional) |
| 1 cup fresh or frozen peas (thawed) | |

Bring 4 quarts of water to a rolling boil. Add the salt and carrots. Boil uncovered for 5 minutes. Add the pasta slowly enough to keep the water boiling. Set the kitchen timer for the amount of time necessary to cook the pasta according to the box. Stir. Slowly add the broccoli when the timer reaches 7 *minutes remaining*. Make sure you add the broccoli slowly enough that the water continues to boil. Stir. Add the peas when there are 4 *minutes remaining*. Drain the pasta and veggies when done and toss with the pesto. Sprinkle with cheese if desired. 4 to 6 servings

*Variation:* Add chopped leftover chicken or nitrite-free ham to complete the meal.

# Homemade Basil Pesto

4 cups packed basil leaves
2 tablespoons pine nuts or walnuts
⅓ cup olive oil
½ teaspoon salt

2 cloves garlic
½ cup (2 ounces) grated Parmesan
cheese

Combine ingredients in a food processor fitted with the steel blade. Process until minced.

*Tip:* Use pesto right a way or place in a small air-tight container and add enough olive oil to cover the top of the pesto and refrigerate up to 2 weeks, or freeze up to 3 months.

## Roasted Summer Veggie Pasta

*Your house is going to smell great while you're cooking this one. Everyone will think you've slaved over it. Once it's in the oven, you can kick up your feet, drink a glass of red wine, and enjoy your family or guests.*

4 bell peppers (red, green, and yellow) diced
1 small eggplant, peeled and diced
2 purple onions, diced
2 small zucchini, diced
3 fresh tomatoes, peeled and diced
4 tablespoons olive oil
1 teaspoon kosher salt
½ teaspoon ground black pepper
½ teaspoon crushed fennel seeds (optional)
8 cups cooked (1 pound) whole-grain pasta
½ cup thinly sliced fresh basil
½ cup freshly grated Parmesan cheese
Additional olive oil for drizzling (optional)

Toss chopped vegetables with olive oil, fennel seeds, salt, and pepper. Line a roasting pan with aluminum foil. Roast veggies in pan at 450 degrees for 1 hour until veggies are tender but not charred. Stir after 30 minutes. Cook pasta during the last 15 minutes of the veggies' cooking time. Drain the pasta and toss with the veggies immediately. Sprinkle with basil and cheese and serve. Drizzle with olive oil if desired. 8 servings

*Variation:* Add roasted sliced chicken, or cooked "hot" or "Italian sweet" nitrite-free turkey or chicken sausage, homemade poultry "sausage"(see Chapter 24), or white beans for protein. Pine nuts make a great garnish.

## Roasted Bell Pepper Pasta

*This quick and easy dish is bursting with flavor and anti-oxidants.*

2 onions, diced
3 cloves garlic, minced
1 tablespoon olive oil
1 (14½-ounce) can diced tomatoes, undrained
1 (24-ounce) jar roasted red bell peppers, sliced in strips
½ teaspoon salt
½ teaspoon ground black pepper
1 tablespoon balsamic vinegar
10 ounces whole-wheat pasta, cooked
½ cup freshly grated Parmesan cheese
½ cup thinly sliced fresh basil *or* 2 teaspoons dried basil
Additional olive oil to drizzle

Cook the onions and garlic in the olive oil in a large nonstick pan over medium heat for 10 minutes, stirring occasionally, until they just start to brown. Add the tomatoes and simmer uncovered for 30 minutes, stirring occasionally. Add the peppers, salt, pepper, and balsamic vinegar. Heat through about 5 minutes. Toss the pasta with the sauce and serve with the basil and cheese. Drizzle with additional olive oil if desired. 6 servings

*Variations:*
- ∾ Add grilled or roasted chicken and mushrooms if desired.
- ∾ For those who don't like chunky sauce, puree the sauce with an emersion blender or in a food processor or blender prior to tossing with the pasta.

# Roasted Winter Veggie Pasta

*This unusual taste combination is robust and flavorful as well as easy and nutritious. I like it with homemade chicken "sausage" that I cook in advance and pull out of the freezer to add to this dish.*

4 cups cubed peeled sweet potato or butternut squash
2 medium onions, diced
2 red bell peppers diced
2 tablespoons olive oil
½ teaspoon salt
½ teaspoon ground black pepper

10 ounces (6 cups) cooked whole-wheat pasta
¼ cup commercial sundried tomato pesto
¼ cup freshly grated Parmesan cheese *or* ¼ cup crumbled feta cheese

Toss cubed sweet potatoes or squash, onions, and bell peppers with olive oil, salt, and pepper. Line a roasting pan with aluminum foil and spray with cooking spray. Roast the veggies in a single layer at 400 degrees for 35 to 45 minutes until the veggies are tender but not charred. Stir once or twice while roasting. Cook pasta during the last few minutes of the veggies' roasting time. Drain the pasta and toss with the roasted veggies and pesto. Sprinkle with cheese. 6 servings

*Variation:* Add cooked Italian turkey or chicken sausage (nitrite-free) or steamed shrimp if desired.

# Herbed Brown Rice

*Fresh herbs are full of antioxidants. Dried herbs are good for you too. You can substitute 2 teaspoons dried herbs for the fresh if they are not available.*

1 large onion, thinly sliced
1 tablespoon olive oil
2 carrots, diced
1 cup brown rice
2 cups water
1 teaspoon salt
½ teaspoon ground black pepper

1 cup fresh parsley, chopped
2 tablespoons mixed fresh herbs, chopped (chives, thyme, oregano, sage, chervil, etc.)
2 cloves garlic, minced
1 tablespoon fresh lemon juice

Cook the onion and carrot in the oil over medium-high heat stirring occasionally for 5 minutes until onion softens. Add the rice, water, and salt. Bring to a boil then reduce to a simmer, covered, for 50 minutes, until water is absorbed. Remove from heat and let rest covered 10 minutes. Stir in the herbs, pepper, garlic, and lemon juice. 4 to 6 servings

*Variation:* Add ½ pound cooked ground chicken or turkey to make "dirty rice."

*Tip:* To chop herbs easily, put them in a measuring cup and snip them with kitchen shears.

# Curried Brown Rice

*This flavorful pilaf is a great accompaniment to chicken or fish dishes.*

1 tablespoon olive oil
1 large onion, thinly sliced
2 cloves garlic, minced
2 carrots, diced or grated
1 tablespoon commercial curry powder
1 teaspoon allspice
1 cup brown basmati rice

2 cups water
1 teaspoon salt
1 cup fresh or frozen peas

*Garnishes:*
½ cup cilantro, chopped (optional)
Cashew nuts
Currants or raisins

Cook the onions, garlic, carrots, and spices in the olive oil in a large pot, over medium heat, stirring occasionally for 5 minutes. Add the water and rice. Bring to a boil, then reduce to a simmer, covered, for 45 minutes. Add the peas and stir. Continue to cook for 5 to 10 more minutes until water is absorbed. Remove from heat and fluff with a fork. Let rest 10 minutes covered. Sprinkle with cilantro, cashews, and currants. 4 to 6 servings

# Millet with Parsley and Lemon

*Millet makes this pilaf light and fluffy. The garlic, lemon, and parsley give it a bright and refreshing taste.*

1 cup millet
2 cups water
1 teaspoon salt
Juice of one lemon

2 cloves of garlic minced
2 tablespoons olive oil
1 cup chopped parsley
½ cup chopped pitted green olives

Cook millet in salted water 20 to 30 minutes until water is absorbed. Toss with lemon juice, garlic, olive oil, olives, and parsley. 4 to 6 servings

*Variation:* Substitute brown rice, bulger, couscous, barley, or quinoa for the millet. Cook the grain according to package directions.

# Lentils and Brown Rice with Caramelized Onions (Megadarra)

*Lentils and brown rice make a complete protein. This delicious dish is a staple in many Mediterranean cultures.*

3 tablespoons olive oil
6 medium yellow onions, thinly sliced
4 cups water
1 cup lentils
1 cup brown rice

1 bay leaf
1 teaspoon salt
½ teaspoon black pepper
¼ cup chopped parsley (optional)
Extra olive oil for drizzling

Heat 3 tablespoons of oil in a large skillet. Add the onions, cover, and cook over medium-low heat for 15 minutes, stirring occasionally, until soft. Uncover the onions, and increase heat to medium. Continue to cook, stirring occasionally, 25 more minutes until golden. Meanwhile, in a large pot, boil the water. Add the rice, bay leaf, and lentils. Simmer covered for 50 minutes until lentils are tender. Add salt and pepper and remove the bay leaf. Serve the rice and lentils with the onions on top. Drizzle a tablespoon of olive oil over each serving (optional) and sprinkle with parsley if desired. 6 servings

# Stir Fried Rice

*This is a less salty, lower-fat alternative to conventional fried rice. Bragg's Liquid Aminos is available in most health food stores and can be used as a seasoning just as you would soy sauce. It has a wonderful flavor and less salt than soy sauce. Unlike soy sauce, it is wheat-free.*

1 cup brown rice
2 cups water
2 teaspoons canola oil
3 carrots, diced or diagonally sliced
1 large onion, diced
6 cloves of garlic, minced
½ small head of cabbage, shredded

1 cup fresh or frozen peas (thawed)
3 tablespoons "lite" soy sauce or
    Bragg's Liquid Aminos
1 tablespoon dark sesame oil
1 teaspoon sugar
2 teaspoons vinegar

Add rice to boiling water, reduce to a simmer, cover, and cook for 50 minutes until water is absorbed. Remove from heat and let stand covered 10 minutes, then fluff with a fork.

Meanwhile, combine the soy sauce, sesame oil, vinegar, and sugar in a small bowl. Set aside. Heat the canola oil in a large frying pan or wok over medium-high heat. Add the onions, garlic, carrots, and cabbage. Cook, stirring constantly for 5 to 7 minutes until vegetables are tender but still crisp. Add the rice, peas, and soy sauce mixture to the vegetables. Stir over medium heat 2 minutes. 4 to 6 servings

*Variations:* Add scrambled eggs, steamed shrimp, cooked cubed chicken, or nitrite-free cubed cooked ham if desired.

# Quick Fruit and Nut Breakfast Pilaf

*This is a great way to start each morning! For around 400 calories you get 30% of your daily calcium, 14 grams of fiber, 21 grams of protein, 20% of your daily iron, and almost a quarter of your vitamin E for the day, not to mention loads of antioxidants and omega-3s. If there is such thing as the perfect breakfast, this may be it!*

½ cup old-fashioned oats
1 cup skim milk or soy milk*
½ cup fresh or frozen blueberries, *or* raspberries, *or* ¼ cup or raisins *or* ¼ cup chopped dried fruit

2 tablespoons ground flaxseed
2 tablespoons wheat germ
2 teaspoons maple syrup (optional)
1 tablespoon toasted walnuts *or* other nuts (optional)

Combine oats, milk, and fruit in a large microwave safe cereal bowl. Microwave on high 3 to 3½ minutes. Stir in flaxseed, wheat germ, and maple syrup if desired. Sprinkle with nuts and enjoy. 1 serving

*When using frozen berries reduce the milk to ¾ cup.

*Variation:* Substitute ½ cup apple sauce *or* cranberry sauce for the fruit and omit the maple syrup.

*Tip:* See how to toast nuts, page 178.

# Protein-Packed Morning Oats

*This is a delicious whole-grain breakfast with enough protein to keep you going all morning. Textured vegetable protein is a soy product that is high in protein and low in fat and carbohydrates. Look for it in the specialty grains and healthfood sections of your supermarket.*

¼ cup whole oats
¼ cup textured vegetable protein
1 cup skim milk

2 tablespoons ground flaxseeds
1 teaspoon maple syrup or honey
(optional)

Place all ingredients from oats through flaxseeds in a microwave safe bowl. Cook on high for 3½ minutes. Let stand 2 to 3 minutes. Add syrup if desired.

# CHAPTER 28

# Healthy and Easy Breads

Few aromas are more enticing than the smell of freshly baked bread. Recently, however, breads have become less popular because so many people are trying to lose weight on low-carb diets. Dieters treat bread like poison. While it's true that it's easy to eat too many calories enjoying breads, they're still a nutritious part of a healthy diet when the breads are made with whole grains and healthy oils.

Nothing is more satisfying than making your own homemade breads, but many feel it takes too much time and effort. However, homemade quick breads, muffins, and pancakes filled with healthy ingredients can be made with just a whisk and a bowl. If you have a bread machine with a dough cycle, you can make excellent quality yeast breads with very little effort or mess. Great whole-grain pizza dough can be made in the food processor or bread machine. Even if you're not a baker, these recipes are simple enough for a novice to get good results. For many it's easier to purchase bread from a reliable baker than to bake breads at home, and that's fine. Just read the label carefully to make sure you are getting 100 percent whole grains and no trans fats.

## Basic Whole-Wheat Bread with Flaxseed

2½ teaspoons of active dry yeast dissolved in 2 tablespoons warm water

1⅓ cup milk (or soy milk)

¼ cup canola oil

¼ cup maple syrup, honey, *or* molasses

3⅓ cups whole-wheat flour such as the King Arthur or Bob's Red Mill brands

½ cup ground flaxseed

1 teaspoon salt

Combine all ingredients in a large bowl and stir until the dough leaves the sides of the bowl. Transfer the dough to a lightly oiled surface, oil your hands, and knead the dough 6 to 8 minutes, until it becomes smooth and elastic. Transfer the dough to a lightly oiled bowl, cover with a towel, and let rise in a warm (about 80 degrees) place for about 60 minutes until the dough is puffy and almost doubled. (Alternatively, the mixing and first rising can be done in a bread machine on dough cycle. I prefer this method.) Transfer the dough to an oiled work surface and shape into an 8-inch log. Place the dough into an 8½ × 4½ inch loaf pan, cover with a towel, and let rise another hour or until it has risen about an inch above the edge of the pan. Preheat the oven to 350 degrees. Bake for 40 minutes, lightly covering it with aluminum foil after the first 20 minutes. The bread is done when tapping on the bottom of the loaf makes a hollow sound.

*Tip:* When you need to roll out or shape dough, put a large sheet of wax paper down on your work surface and oil it or sprinkle it with flour as the recipe directs. When it's time to clean up, you just fold up the wax paper and throw it away. No scrubbing oil, flour, and dough bits up off the counter!

# Whole-Wheat Pizza

*One hundred percent whole-wheat pizza dough may be a little too hearty for many people's taste. Try substituting 1 or 2 cups of white flour for part of the whole-wheat flour if you wish. The trick to good whole-wheat pizza is rolling the dough very thin.*

1 package (2½ teaspoons) active dry yeast
1 teaspoon sugar
1 cup warm water (105 to 115 degrees)

3 cups high quality whole-wheat flour
1 teaspoon kosher salt
1 tablespoon olive oil

Dissolve the yeast and sugar in a small bowl. Combine the flour and salt in the bowl of a food processor fitted with the metal blade. Pulse twice. Add remaining ingredients and process until the mixture forms a ball. Continue processing another minute. Remove the dough from the food processor and knead a few times on a floured surface. Cover the dough and let it rise 30 minutes or more. (You can make the dough in advance and let it rise all day if you wish.) Preheat the oven to 450 degrees. Divide the dough into 2 balls. Place each on a lightly floured surface. Stretch each dough ball carefully into a flat disc then roll the dough with a rolling pin into two 14- to 16-inch circles. Place the dough on a pizza stone or a lightly greased baking sheet and top as desired. Bake at 500 degrees for 12 to 15 minutes (or 450 degrees for 16 to 17 minutes) until crust is lightly browned. Makes 2 14-inch pizzas

*Great easy toppings:* Use traditional pizza sauce and cheese or try basil or sun-dried tomato pesto in place of tomato sauce, feta cheese (a little goes a long way), roasted red bell peppers, very thinly sliced red onion, minced garlic, fresh or dried herbs, and roasted vegetables. Spread pesto on crust, then top with vegetables then cheese.

*Bread machine variation:* Combine all ingredients in the pan of the bread machine in the order recommended by the manufacturer. Process on dough cycle. Remove from pan after the dough cycle is done, let rest 10 minutes and shape and bake as above.

*Technique Tip:* If bread dough is too difficult to work with, knead it a few times (to beat it into submission), and then give it a time-out on your work surface covered with a towel for 10 minutes (to make it truly sorry for thwarting you). After this the dough will be easier to handle.

# Pumpkin Oat Bran Muffins

*Kids love these muffins! They're great for picky eaters. Each muffin has a toddler's serving of vegetables! Three muffins have an adult's serving. Serve them for breakfast with a glass of skim milk or serve them as dessert.*

⅓ cup canola oil
½ cup packed brown sugar
2 eggs
1 (15-ounce) can pumpkin puree
¾ cup whole-wheat flour
   (or sorghum flour)

¾ cup oat bran
1 teaspoon aluminum-free baking
   powder
½ teaspoon salt (optional)
2 teaspoons cinnamon
½ teaspoon allspice

In a large bowl, beat oil, sugar, eggs, and pumpkin with a whisk until well combined. Measure out flour. Add the soda, salt, and spices to the flour in the measuring cup and stir to combine. Add oat bran and flour mixture to the pumpkin mixture. Stir gently until just combined. Do not over stir or the muffins will be tough. Spoon the batter into 12 standard muffin cups lined with paper or sprayed with baking spray. Bake at 350 degrees for 20 to 22 minutes. A toothpick inserted in the center of a muffin should come out clean, but the muffins will be soft. Do not over bake.

*Tip:* Have your muffins or cakes ever turned out tough or heavy? You probably made one of two mistakes: Using a poor quality flour or stirring the batter too much. Using a high quality whole-wheat flour like

King Arthur Brand or Bob's Red Mill brand will give you lighter, tastier baked goods. Having a gentle hand when combining the wet ingredients with the dry will keep your baked goods from being tough. Stir as few times as possible to get the ingredients to come together.

# Peanut Butter Oat Bran Muffins

*This is a tasty variation of the pumpkin oat bran recipe. It's good enough to be a dessert, but each muffin has only 2 teaspoons (8 grams) added sugar. The apples or carrots add sweetness, nutrition, and moistness to the muffins, but the muffins can be made without them.*

¼ cup canola oil

½ cup packed brown sugar

2 eggs

2 apples peeled and grated *or* 2 carrots, finely grated (optional)

½ cup natural peanut butter

¾ cup whole-wheat flour (or sorghum flour)

¾ cup oat bran

1 teaspoon aluminum-free baking powder

½ teaspoon salt (optional)

Beat oil, sugar, eggs, apple, and peanut butter in a medium bowl with a whisk until well combined. Measure out flour. Add the soda and salt to the flour in the measuring cup. Stir to combine. Add the oat bran and the flour mixture to the peanut butter mixture. Stir gently until just combined. Do not over stir or the muffins will be tough. Spoon the batter into 12 standard muffin cups lined with paper or sprayed with baking spray. Bake at 350 degrees for 18 to 20 minutes. A toothpick inserted into the center of a muffin will come out clean. Do not overbake.

*Variation:* For **Banana Peanut Butter Muffins:** Substitute 2 ripe mashed bananas for the apple. Add ½ cup semi-sweet mini chocolate chips.

# Whole-Wheat Muffins (Banana Walnut, Blueberry, Raspberry-Lemon, Cranberry-Orange)

*There are lots of variations for this basic recipe. Just choose your "add-in."*

2 cups whole-wheat flour
½ cup firmly packed brown sugar
⅓ cup canola oil
2 eggs
1 teaspoon vanilla
¾ cup fat-free sour cream or yogurt
1 teaspoon baking soda

Choose one add-in: 2 ripe mashed bananas, 1 teaspoon of cinnamon, and ½ cup chopped walnuts; *or* 2 cups fresh or thawed frozen blueberries; or 2 cups fresh or thawed frozen raspberries and the zest of one organic lemon; or 2 cups chopped cranberries and the zest of an organic orange.

Preheat the oven to 350 degrees. Beat the sugar, oil, eggs, and vanilla with a whisk until well combined. Add the baking soda to the sour cream and stir. It will start to foam.

Combine the flour and baking powder. Gently stir the sour cream mixture and the flour mixture into the sugar mixture. Stir in your choice of add-ins. Stir only until the ingredients are just combined. Stirring too much will make your muffins tough. Spoon into standard muffin cups lined with paper cups or coated with cooking spray. Bake at 350 degrees 20 to 22 minutes. A toothpick inserted into the center of a muffin should come out clean when done. Do not over bake.

*Tip:* Citrus zest is the thin shavings of just the colored part of the fruit's peel (not the bitter white part). Using a tool called a citrus zester is the best way to get the zest, but you can also use a grater with fine holes to get the zest. Always wash the fruit first and use organic fruit whenever possible.

# Whole-Wheat Pancakes (or Waffles)

¾ cup fat-free sour cream, *or* milk, *or* buttermilk, *or* yogurt
1 egg
1 tablespoon canola oil (optional)
1 cup whole-wheat flour or whole-wheat pastry flour

1½ teaspoons aluminum-free baking powder
2 tablespoons ground flaxseed
2 tablespoons wheat germ

Combine sour cream, egg, and oil with a whisk. Stir together remaining ingredients and gently stir them into the sour cream mixture. Do not over mix or the pancakes will be tough. Cook ¼ cup of mixture at a time in a nonstick pan sprayed with cooking spray over medium heat (350 degrees). Flip the pancakes when the tops are covered with bubbles. Makes 8 4-inch pancakes.

*Tip:* Make your own pancake mix: Combine dry ingredients in an airtight container. Just stir into sour cream and egg when you want to cook them.

# Pumpkin Oat Bran Pancakes

¾ cup milk
1 egg
1 cup pumpkin puree (or mashed sweet potato)
1 tablespoon canola oil (optional)
⅔ cup whole-wheat flour

⅔ cup oat bran
1½ teaspoons aluminum-free baking powder
1 teaspoon cinnamon
¼ teaspoon ginger
¼ teaspoon allspice

Combine all ingredients from milk through oil with a whisk. Gently stir in dry ingredients. Do not over mix or your pancakes will be tough. Cook ¼ cup of mixture at a time in a preheated (medium-heat, 350-degree) nonstick pan sprayed with cooking spray. Flip the pancakes when the tops are covered with bubbles. Makes 8 4-inch pancakes.

*Variation:* **Banana Oat Bran Pancakes:** Substitute 1 ripe mashed banana for the pumpkin.

# Fluffy Oat Waffles or Pancakes (wheat-free)

*The soy flower adds protein to these pancakes. You can find soy flour in most large supermarkets and health food stores. If you like, you can substitute ¼ cup ground flaxseeds or ¼ cup more oats for the soy flour. The ricotta cheese makes the pancakes light and fluffy.*

1 cup old-fashioned oats
¼ cup soy flour
1½ teaspoons aluminum-free baking powder
1 teaspoon canola oil

1 egg plus one egg white
⅔ cup milk
¼ cup part-skim ricotta cheese *or* ¼ cup low-fat small curd cottage cheese

Combine all ingredients until just mixed. Cook ¼ cup of mixture at a time in a preheated waffle iron or a (medium-heat, 350-degree) nonstick pan sprayed with cooking spray. Flip the pancakes when the tops are covered with bubbles.

# Pita Chips

Cut each pita into 8 wedges. Split the wedges open. Spread the triangles out on a baking sheet in a single layer. Bake at 350 degrees for 10 to 15 minutes, until crisp. Drizzle with olive oil or spray with cooking spray, then sprinkle with salt or seasoned salt if desired. Store in an airtight container once they're cool.

# Whole-Grain Croutons

Cut whole-grain bread into 1-inch cubes. Spray with cooking spray or drizzle with olive oil and sprinkle with salt and garlic powder if desired. Bake at 350 degrees, stirring once, for 10 to 15 minutes until crunchy. Store in an airtight container when cool.

# Easy Baked French Toast

6 slices whole-grain bread
¼ cup wheat germ (optional)
6 eggs, beaten
1 cup skim milk
1 teaspoon vanilla or almond extract

Optional spices (add any or all):
½ teaspoon ginger, ½ teaspoon
cinnamon, ½ teaspoon nutmeg,
zest of an organic orange or lemon

Rip bread into 1-inch chunks and place in a 9 × 9-inch baking dish sprayed with cooking spray. Whisk together remaining ingredients and pour them over the bread. Refrigerate to allow the bread to soak up the mixture for 15 minutes or overnight. Bake at 350 degrees 15 to 20 minutes. Serve with powdered sugar, maple syrup, or honey if desired. 6 servings

---

### Savvy Eating Tip: Food Allergies

Those with a milk allergy can freely substitute the same amount of soy or rice milk for the skim milk in these recipes. Soy yogurt and sour cream, however, will not give as good results when substituted for the dairy versions.

Those with wheat allergy or gluten sensitive enteropathy (Celiac disease) can substitute sorghum or teff, an African grain, flour for the same amount of whole-wheat flour in the bread and dessert recipes that don't use yeast. (Ask your grocer to order them from Bob's Red Mill if you can't find them where you shop.)

Those with egg allergies can use egg-free substitutes in most baked goods. In general, the finished product will not rise as high or be as rich. Shop for egg-free substitutes at health food stores or online at ener-g.com, or make your own.

- For each egg substitute: 1 teaspoon baking powder, 1 table-spoon water, and 1 tablespoon vinegar or
- For each egg substitute: 1 teaspoon baking powder, 1½ tea-spoons of oil, and 1½ teaspoons water

Consult The Food Allergy and Anaphylaxis Network at www.food allergy.org for more recipe and substitution ideas as well as lots of excellent information on avoiding allergens in foods.

Before giving up a healthy food in your diet, consult a physician to make sure you do have an allergy.

If you do have a food allergy, be sure to carry an epi-pen (prescribed by your doctor) for emergencies.

# CHAPTER 29

# Soothe Your Sweet Tooth with Better Treats

Desserts are certainly not necessary nutritionally, but for some of us they're important psychologically. They give us a sense of celebration and indulgence. Desserts can be healthy and sweet like a bowl of fresh fruit or dripping with saturated fat and sugar like a frosted cake. Rich, sweet, heavy desserts can often be replaced with healthier choices, but the alternative needs to be as tasty and satisfying as the traditional dessert. If you crave turtle cheesecake, a nice bowl of strawberries isn't going to cut it no matter how delicious they are.

However, I've found that the desserts that are the sweetest or the richest aren't necessarily the best tasting. I've also found that it's not too much to ask of your dessert to give your body something it needs. For example, most baked goods like cookies, cakes, and brownies taste great when made with whole-grain flour or with added whole grains. Healthy nuts and fruits make excellent additions to cookies, cakes, and pies.

These dessert recipes have been modified to eliminate trans fats and limit saturated fats. They're also lower in sugar than traditional sweets. Decreasing the sugar while adding ingredients like whole grains, nuts, and peanut butter decreases the dessert's GI without decreasing satisfaction.

Make no mistake; even these desserts are not health food. You would be better off nutritionally if you avoided sweets entirely, but most of us aren't willing to go that far. The following recipes are designed to *replace* less healthy desserts already in your diet. It is still necessary to limit portion size.

# Fruit Smoothie

*To get semi-frozen fruit either place chopped fruit in a single layer in the freezer for 30 minutes, or thaw frozen fruit at room temperature for 30 minutes, or thaw briefly in the microwave (times vary).*

2 cups semi-frozen fruit (berries, peaches, mango, etc.)
1 cup low-fat or fat-free plain yogurt *plus* 2 tablespoons honey or sugar

*or*
1 cup low-fat or fat-free vanilla yogurt

Place all ingredients in a blender and process until blended.

# Fruit Ice

*This fruit ice is bursting with flavor because it doesn't contain lots of added water, corn syrup, or artificial sweeteners like most commercial ices. Honey has a lower glycemic load than sugar or corn syrup, so it's the preferred sweetener.*

2 cups semi-frozen fruit (berries, peaches, mango, cantaloupe, seeded watermelon)

2 tablespoons lemon juice
1 tablespoon honey or sugar to taste (optional)

Place all ingredients in blender and process until blended. Add water or fruit juice a tablespoon at a time if too thick to blend. 2 servings

# Yogurt Cream

*Draining the yogurt produces a thick, rich-tasting, creamy yogurt with less sour tanginess than typical yogurt. You can enjoy it unsweetened or add an artificial sweetener in place of the honey.*

16 ounces fat-free or low-fat plain natural yogurt

1 to 3 teaspoons honey, maple syrup, *or* sugar to taste
¼ teaspoon vanilla

Place a sieve or colander in a large bowl. Line the colander with a paper coffee filter or a double thickness of paper towels. Spoon the yogurt into the filter. Cover and place in the refrigerator for 2 to 8 hours. Discard the liquid in the bowl. Scrape the yogurt cream off the filter into a bowl and stir in honey and vanilla. Enjoy with fruit or use in place of whipped cream. 2 servings

*Variations:* Substitute 16 ounces skim or part-skim ricotta cheese for the yogurt. No need to drain the ricotta. Substitute almond extract for the vanilla. Substitute 1 tablespoon of fruit jam for the honey.

# Kids' Favorite Banana Sundaes

1 banana
6 ounces vanilla or other flavor non-fat yogurt or yogurt cream
1 tablespoon chocolate syrup

1 tablespoon roasted, lightly salted peanuts, almonds, or sunflower seeds
1 teaspoon sprinkles or mini chocolate chips (optional)

Chop banana into a bowl. Add remaining ingredients. 2 servings

# Flourless Peanut Butter Cookies

*These delicate tasty cookies have ½ the sugar of conventional peanut butter cookies.*

1 cup all natural peanut butter
¼ cup packed brown sugar
1 egg
1 teaspoon aluminum-free baking powder

1 teaspoon vanilla
3 tablespoons white sugar (optional)

Cream together all ingredients. Scoop up rounded teaspoonfuls of dough, form them into a ball, and roll them in the sugar (optional). Place the dough balls on an ungreased cookie sheet and flatten slightly. Bake at 350 for 10 minutes. Cookies will be soft, and not brown. Cool on a wire rack. 40 cookies

*Tip:* Make small (1 teaspoon-sized) cookies. You're less likely to over indulge if the cookie size is smaller.

# Double Chocolate Cookies

*These deep dark chocolate cookies are so satisfying!*

½ cup canola oil
½ cup brown sugar *or* honey
1 egg
1 teaspoon vanilla
1 cup whole-wheat flour
⅓ cup cocoa powder

1 teaspoon aluminum-free baking
    powder
¼ teaspoon salt (optional)
1 cup chocolate chips
¾ cup walnut pieces (optional)

In a large bowl, whisk together all ingredients from canola oil through vanilla. Add the flour, cocoa powder, baking powder, and salt and stir gently until just combined. Stir in chocolate chips and nuts. Drop by rounded teaspoonfuls on to an ungreased baking sheet. Bake at 375 degrees for 8 to 10 minutes, until set but still soft.

# Oatmeal Spice Cookies

*These wholesome cookies have ⅓ less sugar than typical oatmeal cookies, but twice the flavor. They're also packed full of whole grains.*

Whisk together oil through vanilla in a large bowl until well combined. Add all the ingredients from the flour through the oats. Stir gently to combine. Stir in walnuts and raisins if desired. Drop teaspoonfuls of dough onto an ungreased cookie sheet, bake at 350 degrees for 8 minutes until lightly browned but still soft. Do not overbake. 2 dozen

⅓ cup canola oil
⅓ cup of dark brown sugar, packed
1 egg
2 teaspoons vanilla
¾ cup whole-wheat flour (substitute
    ¾ cup millet or sorghum flour if
    desired)
½ teaspoon aluminum-free baking
    powder

¼ teaspoon salt (optional)
½ teaspoon cinnamon
¼ teaspoon allspice
¼ teaspoon ground ginger
1½ cups of old-fashioned oats
½ cup chopped walnuts (optional)
½ cup raisins (optional)

# Almond Cake

*This rich cake has ⅓ less sugar than the traditional cake and is made with canola oil rather than butter and whole-wheat pastry flour (Bob's Red Mill brand is a quality brand and is widely available in grocery stores.) It's similar to a pound cake with the goodness of almonds.*

1 cup almonds
¾ cup sugar
¾ cup canola oil
1 teaspoon vanilla
1 teaspoon almond extract

5 eggs (or 2 eggs and 6 egg whites)
1 cup whole-wheat pastry flour
1½ teaspoons aluminum-free baking
  powder
¼ teaspoon salt

Place almonds in food processor equipped with a chopping blade. Process until the almonds are finely ground. Add the sugar, oil, vanilla, almond extract, and eggs. Process until well mixed. Add the dry ingredients to the almond mixture. Pulse the processor 3 times until combined. Do not over mix. Pour batter into a 13 × 9-inch pan lined with parchment or waxed paper and sprayed with vegetable oil cooking spray. Bake at 325 for 35 minutes until a toothpick inserted in the center comes out clean. When cool, slice into12 3-inch squares. Slice the squares diagonally into triangles (like baklava). Garnish with a dusting of powdered sugar and fresh fruit if desired. 12–24 servings

# Amaretti Cookies

*These Old World cookies are much less sweet than American favorites, but have a rich satisfying taste and a heavenly aroma when baking. Serve these with dried apricots for a healthy dessert alternative.*

1 pound whole almonds
⅓ cup confectioner's sugar
2 teaspoons vanilla

2 egg whites
½ teaspoon cardamom (optional)

Place the almonds in the bowl of a food processor fitted with the chopping blade. Process until finely ground. Add the sugar, vanilla, egg, and cardamom to the ground almonds. Process until well mixed. Drop dough by rounded teaspoonfuls onto a baking sheet sprayed with cooking spray. Bake at 350 degrees for 15 minutes until lightly browned. 50 cookies

# Chocolate Zucchini Cake

*The zucchini adds moisture to the cake, but it's optional.*

1½ cups sugar
1¾ cups whole-wheat flour*
¾ cup cocoa
1½ teaspoons baking soda
1½ teaspoons aluminum-free baking powder
1 teaspoon salt

2 eggs
1 cup skim milk
½ cup canola oil
2 teaspoons vanilla
1 cup boiling water
2 cups grated zucchini (peeling is optional)

Combine all the ingredients from the sugar through the salt in a large bowl. Add eggs, milk, oil, and vanilla and beat with an electric mixer 2 minutes. Stir in the boiling water. The mixture will be thin. Pour the batter into a greased 13 × 9-inch cake pan and bake at 350 degrees for 38 to 42 minutes until toothpick inserted into the center comes out clean.

*Tip:* Frost for special occasions with peanut butter or chocolate frosting or top with ½ cup chocolate chips and ½ cup chopped nuts while still warm. The cake can be baked in 2 8-inch round cake pans for 25 minutes.

*You can make this cake **gluten free** by substituting teff flour or sorghum flour for the whole wheat. Look for these flours at health food stores that carry Bob's Red Mill brand.

# Apple Cake

*This is a family favorite with half the sugar of the traditional cake.*

1 cup canola oil
1 cup sugar *or* ⅔ cup honey
3 eggs
3 cups peeled apples, grated or chopped
1 teaspoon vanilla

3 cups whole-wheat flour
1 teaspoon salt (optional)
1 teaspoon aluminum-free baking powder
3 teaspoons cinnamon
1 cup chopped pecans (optional)

Combine oil through vanilla and beat well. Stir in remaining ingredients until just combined. Pour batter into a tube pan coated with cooking spray. Bake at 325 degrees for 50 to 60 minutes, until a toothpick inserted into the center comes out clean.

*Variations:* Serve with *caramel glaze* for special occasions: Combine 4 tablespoons butter, ⅓ cup brown sugar, and 2 tablespoons of milk in a sauce pan. Bring to a boil then simmer for 2½ minutes. Pour over cake while it is still warm.

*Banana Cake:* Substitute 3 mashed bananas for the apple.

*Zucchini Cake:* Substitute 3 cups grated zucchini for the apples.

# Berry Crisp

⅔ cup sugar
1 16-ounce package frozen
  blueberries*
1 16-ounce package frozen
  raspberries*
1 16-ounce package frozen cherries*
¼ cup whole-wheat flour
¼ teaspoon salt (optional)
2 tablespoons chilled trans-fat-free
  margarine *or* butter cut into
  small pieces

4 tablespoons brown sugar
¼ cup whole-wheat flour
  (or millet flour)
¼ cup old-fashioned oats
1½ teaspoons cinnamon
2 tablespoons sliced almonds *or*
  pecans (optional)

Combine sugar, berries, flour, and salt in a 13 × 9-inch pan coated with cooking spray. Combine butter through cinnamon in a medium bowl, until the mixture is combined but still lumpy. Sprinkle butter mixture over fruit. Sprinkle with nuts. Bake at 400 degrees for 40 minutes.

*If using fresh fruit, decrease the flour in the fruit mixture to 2 tablespoons and decrease baking time to 30 minutes.

*Variations:* Substitute cranberries or other combinations of berries for the ones in the recipe or substitute a pound of *grated* apple for any one of the berries.

## Crustless Pumpkin Streusel Pie

*The crust is usually the most unhealthy part of the pie. In this pie, the crust is replaced by a lighter, flaky streusel.*

⅓ cup honey, maple syrup, or sugar
½ teaspoon salt
1 teaspoon cinnamon
½ teaspoon ground ginger
¼ teaspoon ground allspice
2 eggs
1 (15-ounce) can pumpkin puree

½ cup skim milk
3 tablespoons brown sugar
2 tablespoons whole-wheat flour
1½ teaspoons cinnamon
2 tablespoons chilled butter cut into small pieces

In a large bowl, whisk together all the ingredients from the sugar through the milk. Pour mixture into a deep 9-inch pie pan that has been sprayed with cooking spray. Combine remaining ingredients in a medium bowl. Mix until the lumps are the size of small peas. Sprinkle sugar mixture over pumpkin mixture. Bake at 350 degrees for 40 to 50 minutes, until a knife inserted into the center comes out clean.

*Variation:* You can substitute 2 teaspoons pumpkin pie spice for the cinnamon, ginger, and allspice.

## Whole-Wheat Brownies

*These whole-wheat brownies have ¼ less sugar than typical brownies. My son likes them even better than conventional brownies because the deep chocolate flavor comes through when the brownie is less sweet.*

⅔ cup canola oil
1½ cup brown sugar
2 teaspoons vanilla
4 eggs
¾ cup cocoa powder
1 teaspoon aluminum-free baking powder

2 teaspoons vinegar
1 teaspoon instant coffee granules (optional)
1 cup whole-wheat flour
1 cup chocolate chips (optional)
1 cup chopped walnuts (optional)

Combine oil through coffee and mix thoroughly. Gently stir in flour. Pour into a greased 13 × 9-inch pan. Bake at 350 for 20 to 25 minutes.

(Alternatively, use a 10 × 15-inch jellyroll pan and bake for 18 to 22 minutes.) Cut into 1½-inch squares. Makes 48.

*Variation:* Aztec brownies. Add 1 teaspoon cinnamon and 1 teaspoon chili powder with the dry ingredients. These spicy brownies are even better than the original recipe. Serve hot with a scoop of vanilla ice cream or frozen yogurt.

# BIBLIOGRAPHY

Atzmon G, Yang XM, Muzumdar R, et al. Differential gene expression between visceral and subcutaneous fat depots. *Horm Metab Res* (Germany), Nov-Dec 2002; 34(11–12) p622–8.

Baranowska B, Chmielowska M, Wolinska-Witort E, et al. The relationship between neuropeptides and hormones in starvation. *Neuro Endocrinol Lett* (Sweden), Oct 2001; 22(5) p349–55.

Bell SJ, Sears B. Low-glycemic-load diets: impact on obesity and chronic diseases. *Crit Rev Food Sci Nutr* (United States), 2003; 43(4) p357–77.

Bjorntorp P. Metabolic difference between visceral fat and subcutaneous abdominal fat. *Diabetes Metab* (France), Jun 2000; 26 Suppl 3 p10–2.

Brand-Miller JC, Thomas M, Swan V, et al. Physiological validation of the concept of glycemic load in lean young adults. *J Nutr* (United States), Sep 2003; 133(9) p2728–32.

Brand-Miller, JC, and PK. Foster. Diets with Low Glycemic Index: From Theory to Practice. *Nutrition Today*, 1999; 34 p64–72.

Briefel RR, Reidy K, Karwe V, et al. Toddlers' transition to table foods: Impact on nutrient intakes and food patterns. *J Am Diet Assoc* (United States), Jan 2004; 104(1 Suppl 1) ps38–44.

Brown R, Ogden J. Children's eating attitudes and behaviour: a study of the modelling and control theories of parental influence. *Health Educ Res* (England), Jun 2004; 19(3) p261–71.

Cardador-Martinez A, Loarca-Pina G, Oomah BD. Antioxidant activity in common beans (Phaseolus vulgaris L.) *J Agric Food Chem* (United States), Nov 20 2002; 50(24) p6975–80.

Carper JL, Orlet Fisher J, Birch LL. Young girls' emerging dietary restraint and disinhibition are related to parental control in child feeding. *Appetite* (England), Oct 2000; 35(2) p121–9.

Floyd H. Chilton, Ph.D., *Inflammation Nation* (New York: Simon and Schuster, 2005).

Clasey, JL, Weltman, Patrie, Weltman, Pezzolis, Bouchard, Thorner, Hartman. Visceral fat and fasting insulin greatest predictors of 24 hour GH concentrations. *J. Clinical Endocrinol Metab.* 2001 Aug; 86 (8): p3485–52.

Cnop M, Landchild MJ, Vidal J, et al. The concurrent accumulation of intra-abdominal and subcutaneous fat explains the association between insulin resistance and plasma leptin concentrations : distinct metabolic effects of two fat compartments. *Diabetes* (United States), Apr 2002; 51(4) p1005–15.

Cordain, Loren. *The Paleo Diet: Lose Weight and Get Healthy by Eating the Food You Were Designed to Eat* (Wiley, 2001).

Dewey, KG. Is breastfeeding protective against child obesity? *J Hum Lact* (United States), Feb 2003; 19(1) p9–18.

Drapeau V, Therrien F, Richard D, et al. Is visceral obesity a physiological adaptation to stress? *Panminerva Med* (Italy), Sep 2003; 45(3) p189–95.

Eades, M.R., and M. D. Eades, *Protein Power: The High-Protein/Low-Carbohydrate Way to Lose Weight, Feel Fit, and Boost Your Health—In Just Weeks*, (Bantam Books, 1999).

Fisher FM, McTernan PG, Valsamakis G, et al. Differences in adiponectin protein expression: effect of fat depots and type 2 diabetic status. *Horm Metab Res* (Germany), Nov-Dec 2002; 34(11–12) p650–4.

Faith MS, Keller KL, Johnson SL, et al. Familial aggregation of energy intake in children. *Am J Clin Nutr* (United States), May 2004; 79(5) p844–50.

FDA—Mercury Levels in Commercial Fish and Shellfish. http://vm.cfsan.fda.gov/~frf/sea-mehg.html.

Fisher JO, Mitchell DC, Smiciklas-Wright H, et al. Parental influences on young girls' fruit and vegetable, micronutrient, and fat intakes. *J Am Diet Assoc* (United States), Jan 2002; 102(1) p58–64.

Frank L, Marian A, Visser M, et al. Exposure to peanuts in utero and in infancy and the development of sensitization to peanut allergens in young children. *Pediatr Allergy Immunol* (Denmark), Feb 1999; 10(1) p27–32.

Fisher JO, Mitchell DC, Smiciklas-Wright H, et al. Parental influences on young girls' fruit and vegetable, micronutrient, and fat intakes. *J Am Diet Assoc* (United States), Jan 2002; 102(1) p58–64.

French SA, Harnack L, Jeffery RW. Fast food restaurant use among women in the Pound of Prevention study: dietary, behavioral and demographic correlates. *Int J Obes Relat Metab Disord* (England), Oct 2000; 24(10) p1353–9.

Gannon, MC, F.Q. Nuttall, Westphal, S. Fang, N. Ercan-Fang. Acute Metabolic Response to high-carb, high starch meals compared with moderate-carb, low-starch meals in subjects with type 2 diabetes. *Diabetes Care*, Oct 21, 1998; (10) p1619–26.

Gong H, Ni Y, Guo X, et al. Resistin promotes 3T3-L1 preadipocyte differentiation. *Eur J Endocrinol* (England), Jun 2004; 150(6) p885–92.

Hoppin, Allison G. Assesment and Management of Childhood Obesity. *Medscape*. 2004. http://www.medscape.com/viewprogram/3221.

Herbert, Victor and G. Subak-Sharpe, *Total Nutrition* (St. Martin's Press, 1995).

Hu, FB, et al. Frequent Nut Consumption and Risk of Coronary Heart Disease in Women: Prospective Cohort Study. *British Medical Journal* (1998); 317 p1341–45.

Huang XF, Xin X, McLennan P, et al. Role of fat amount and type in ameliorating diet-induced obesity: insights at the level of hypothalamic arcuate nucleus leptin receptor, neuropeptide Y and pro-opiomelanocortin mRNA expression. *Diabetes Obes Metab* (England), Jan 2004; 6(1) p35–44.

Jang Y, Kim OY, Ryu HJ, et al. Visceral fat accumulation determines postprandial lipemic response, lipid peroxidation, DNA damage, and endothelial dysfunction in nonobese Korean men. *J Lipid Res* (United States), Dec 2003; 44(12) p2356–64.

Jensdottir T, Arnadottir IB, Thorsdottir I, et al. Relationship between dental erosion, soft drink consumption, and gastroesophageal reflux among Icelanders. *Clin Oral Investig* (Germany), Jun 2004; 8(2) p91–6.

Johnston CS, Taylor CA, Hampl JS. More Americans are eating "5 a day" but intakes of dark green and cruciferous vegetables remain low. *J Nutr* (United States), Dec 2000; 130(12) p3063–7.

Johnson RK. Changing eating and physical activity patterns of US children. *Proc Nutr Soc* (England), May 2000; 59(2) p295–301.

Kant AK, Graubard BI. Eating out in America, 1987–2000: trends and nutritional correlates. *Prev Med* (United States), Feb 2004; 38(2) p243–9.

Kim MS, Namkoong C, Kim HS, et al. Chronic central administration of ghrelin reverses the effects of leptin. *Int J Obes Relat Metab Disord* (England), Oct 2004; 28(10) p1264–71.

Kurioka S, Murakami Y, Nishiki M, et al. Relationship between visceral fat accumulation and anti-lipolytic action of insulin in patients with type 2 diabetes mellitus. *Endocr J* (Japan), Aug 2002; 49(4) p459–64.

Kozlowska-Wojciechowska M, Uramowska-Zyto B, Jarosz A, et al. Impact of school children's nutrition education program on the knowledge and nutritional behavior of their parents. *Rocz Panstw Zakl Hig* (Poland), 2002; 53(3) p253–8 (Abstract).

Krahnstoever Davison K, Lipps Birch L. Obesigenic families: parents' physical activity and dietary intake patterns predict girls' risk of overweight. *Int J Obes Relat Metab Disord* (England), Sep 2002; 26(9) p1186–93.

Kris-Etherton PM, Keen CL. Evidence that the antioxidant flavonoids in tea and cocoa are beneficial for cardiovascular health. *Curr Opin Lipidol* (England), Feb 2002; 13(1) p41–9.

Kleinman, R. D., *Pediatric Nutrition Handbook*, 5th ed. (American Academy of Pediatrics, 2004).

Laessle RG, Uhl H, Lindel B, et al. Parental influences on laboratory eating behavior in obese and non-obese children. *Int J Obes Relat Metab Disord* (England), May 2001; 25 Suppl 1 pS60–2.

Laitinen J, Pietilainen K, Wadsworth M, et al. Predictors of abdominal obesity among 31-y-old men and women born in Northern Finland in 1966. *Eur J Clin Nutr* (England), Jan 2004; 58(1) p180–90.

Lim GP, Chu T, Yang F, et al. The curry spice curcumin reduces oxidative damage and amyloid pathology in an Alzheimer transgenic mouse. *J Neurosci* (United States), Nov 1 2001; 21(21) p8370–7.

Liu S, Manson JE, Lee IM, et al. Fruit and vegetable intake and risk of cardiovascular disease: the Women's Health Study. *Am J Clin Nutr* (United States), Oct 2000; 72(4) p922–8.

Liuzzi A, Savia G, Tagliaferri M, et al. Serum leptin concentration in moderate and severe obesity: relationship with clinical, anthropometric and metabolic factors. *Int J Obes Relat Metab Disord* (England), Oct 1999; 23(10) p1066–73.

Ludwig DS, Ebbeling CB. Type 2 diabetes mellitus in children: primary care and public health considerations. *JAMA* (United States), Sep 26 2001; 286(12) p1427–30.

Marniemi J, Kronholm E, Aunola S, et al. Visceral fat and psychosocial stress in identical twins discordant for obesity. *J Intern Med* (England), Jan 2002; 251(1) p35–43.

McBean LD, Miller GD. Enhancing the nutrition of America's youth. *J Am Coll Nutr* (United States), Dec 1999; 18(6) p563–71.

McCrory MA, Fuss PJ, Hays NP, et al. Overeating in America: association between restaurant food consumption and body fatness in healthy adult men and women ages 19 to 80. *Obes Res* (United States), Nov 1999; 7(6) p564–71.

Michaud DS, Liu S, Giovannucci E, et al. Dietary sugar, glycemic load, and pancreatic cancer risk in a prospective study. *J Natl Cancer Inst* (United States), Sep 4 2002; 94(17) p1293–300.

National Diabetes Statistics. http://diabetes.niddk.nih.gov/dm/pubs/statistics.

Nakamura Y, Okamura T, Tamaki S, et al. Egg consumption, serum cholesterol, and cause-specific and all-cause mortality: the National Integrated Project for Prospective Observation of Non-communicable Disease and Its Trends in the Aged, 1980 (NIPPON DATA80). *Am J Clin Nutr* (United States), Jul 2004; 80(1) p58–63.

National Heart, Lung and Blood Institute (NHLBI), Obesity Guidelines-Executive Summary-BMI Chart http://www.nhlbi.nih.gov/guidelines/obesity/bmi_tbl.htm.

Nestle, M, and Jacobson. Halting the Obesity epidemic: A public health policy approach. *Public Health Reports* (2000); 115 p12–24.

Nicklas TA, Elkasabany A, Srinivasan SR, et al. Trends in nutrient intake of 10-year-old children over two decades (1973–1994) : the Bogalusa Heart Study. *Am J Epidemiol* (United States), May 15 2001; 153(10) p969–77.

Neuhouser ML, Patterson RE, Thornquist MD, et al. Fruits and vegetables are associated with lower lung cancer risk only in the placebo arm of the beta-carotene and retinol efficacy trial (CARET). *Cancer Epidemiol Biomarkers Prev* (United States), Apr 2003; 12(4) p350–8.

Northstone K, Emmett P, Nethersole F. The effect of age of introduction to lumpy solids on foods eaten and reported feeding difficulties at 6 and 15 months. *J Hum Nutr Diet* (England), Feb 2001; 14(1) p43–54.

Ogden, CL, Flegal KM, Carol MD,Johnson CL. Prevalence and trends in overweight among US children and adolescents, 1999–2000. JAMA 2002: 288:1728–1732.

Orlet Fisher J, Rolls BJ, Birch LL. Children's bite size and intake of an entree are greater with large portions than with age-appropriate or self-selected portions. *Am J Clin Nutr* (United States), May 2003; 77(5) p1164–70.

Oomen CM, Ocke MC, Feskens EJ, et al. Association between trans fatty acid intake and 10-year risk of coronary heart disease in the Zutphen Elderly Study: a prospective population-based study. *Lancet* (England), Mar 10 2001; 357(9258) p746–51.

Pasquali R, Vicennati V. Activity of the hypothalamic-pituitary-adrenal axis in different obesity phenotypes. *Int J Obes Relat Metab Disord* (England), Jun 2000; 24 Suppl 2 pS47–9.

Rajala MW, Qi Y, Patel HR, et al. Regulation of resistin expression and circulating levels in obesity, diabetes, and fasting. *Diabetes* (United States), Jul 2004; 53(7) p1671–9.

Rask-Nissila L, Jokinen E, Terho P, et al. Effects of diet on the neurologic development of children at 5 years of age: the STRIP project. *J Pediatr* (United States), Mar 2002; 140(3) p328–33.

Rolls BJ, Morris EL, Roe LS. Portion size of food affects energy intake in normal-weight and overweight men and women. *Am J Clin Nutr* (United States), Dec 2002; 76(6) p1207–13.

Rolls BJ, Ello-Martin JA, Tohill BC. What can intervention studies tell us about the relationship between fruit and vegetable consumption and weight management? *Nutr Rev* (United States), Jan 2004; 62(1) p1–17.

de Roos NM, Bots ML, Katan MB. Replacement of dietary saturated fatty acids by trans fatty acids lowers serum HDL cholesterol and impairs endothelial function in healthy men and women. *Arterioscler Thromb Vasc Biol* (United States), Jul 2001; 21(7) p1233–7.

Satter, Ellyn, *Child of Mine: Feeding With Love and Good Sense* (Bull Publishing Company, 2000).

Slattery ML, Benson J, Ma KN, et al. Trans-fatty acids and colon cancer. *Nutr Cancer* (United States), 2001; 39(2) p170–5.

Soriguer F, Moreno F, Rojo-Martinez G, et al. Redistribution of abdominal fat after a period of food restriction in rats is related to the type of dietary fat. *Br J Nutr* (England), Jan 2003; 89(1) p115–22.

Southon S. Increased fruit and vegetable consumption: potential health benefits. *Nutr Metab Cardiovasc Dis* (Italy), Aug 2001; 11(4 Suppl) p78–81.

Spencer, JW, and J Jacobs, *Complementary and Alternative Medicine: An Evidence-Based Approach* (Mosby, 2003).

Tseng M. The influence of the parent on childhood dietary intake. *Public Health Nutr* (England), Apr 2004; 7(2) p251–2.

USDA Nutrient Database 17, 2005. http://www.nal.usda.gov/fnic/foodcomp/Data/SR17/sr17.html.

Vinson JA, Mandarano M, Hirst M, et al. Phenol antioxidant quantity and quality in foods: beers and the effect of two types of beer on an animal model of atherosclerosis. *J Agric Food Chem* (United States), Aug 27 2003; 51(18) p5528–33.

Wadden TA, Butryn ML. Behavioral treatment of obesity. *Endocrinol Metab Clin North Am* (United States), Dec 2003; 32(4) p981–1003.

Weil, Andrew, *Natural Health, Natural Medicine* (Houghton Mifflin, 1995).

Wittaker RC, Wright JA, Pepe MS, Seidel KD, Deitz WH. Predicting obesity in young adulthood from childhood and adult obesity. *N Engl J Med*, 1997; 337 p869–873.

Wideman, L, JY Weltman, ML Hartman, Veldhuis, Weltman. GH release during acute and chronic aerobic and resistance exercise. *Sports Med*, 2002; 32(15) p987–1004.

Willett, WC. *Eat, Drink, and Be Healthy* (Simon and Schuster, 2001).

Willett, WC, et al. Is Dietary Fat a Major Determinant of Body Fat? *American Journal of Clinical Nutrition*, 1998; 67 p556–62.

Wolfe, BM, and LA Pische. Replacement of Carbohydrate by Protein in a Conventional-fat Diet Reduces Triglyceride Concentrations in Healthy Normolipidemic Subjects. *Clinical and Investigational Medicine*, 1999; 22 p140–48.

Worobey J. Early family mealtime experiences and eating attitudes in normal weight, underweight and overweight females. *Eat Weight Disord* (Italy), Mar 2002; 7(1) p39–44.

Wyshak G. Teenaged girls, carbonated beverage consumption, and bone fractures. *Arch Pediatr Adolesc Med* (United States), Jun 2000; 154(6) p610–3.

Yip I, Go VL, Hershman JM, et al. Insulin-leptin-visceral fat relation during weight loss. *Pancreas* (United States), Aug 2001; 23(2) p197–203.

Young LR, Nestle M. The contribution of expanding portion sizes to the US obesity epidemic. *Am J Public Health* (United States), Feb 2002; 92(2) p246–9.

# Recipe Index

# INDEX

*Recipes are included in a separate index.*